GHOST
MOUNTAIN
BOOKS

The Dubrow Diet

Interval Eating to
Lose Weight and Feel Ageless

by

Heather Dubrow
&
Terry Dubrow M.D., F.A.C.S.

GHOST
MOUNTAIN
BOOKS

Published in Los Angeles, California, by Ghost Mountain Books, Inc.

ISBN:

Print: 9781939457714

EPUB: 9781939457721

Mobi: 9781939457738

Jacket photo: Rod Foster/Gigasavvy.com

Jacket design: Alina Baloi

Interior design and production: Dovetail Publishing Services

Dedications

I dedicate this book to my incredibly shredded husband (he asked me to write that—ha ha). Our journey to a life of healthy eating, exercise, and a positive body image has been fun, crazy, difficult, and rewarding. Thank you for giving me the gift of an ageless body, mind, and soul. I love you, Honyi!

I dedicate this book to my incredible wife, who taught me how to eat healthfully while still keeping it delicious and fun. No textbook, scientific literature, or nutritional guide has taught me as much about how to feel your best, lose weight, and still enjoy yourself as much as Heather has. This game-changing book is because of you, Honyi, and I'm more grateful every day that I get to live with you, love you, and be a part of your amazing world.

Contents

Acknowledgments

This book is very special and personal to us, and we are so lucky to have the team we have standing with us. Thank you to our children, Nicky, Max, Kat, and Coco; we love you so much, and we hope we are giving you a positive and appropriate view of living the healthiest life through proper eating and exercise.

Thank you to everyone at Ghost Mountain books! Jay McGraw, Lisa Clark, Andrea McKinnon, and Carly Stratton: we are eternally grateful for your support and understanding of our cutting-edge diet plan. Gretchen Lees: you are the hippest, coolest, smartest, funniest gal on the planet, and we are so lucky to have you in our world. And to Julia Serebrinsky—thank you for sharing your impressive culinary creativity and skill with us.

Thank you to our agents Lance Klein, Mel Berger, Ryan McNeily, and Justin Ongert at WME for always supporting us!

Finally, thank you to the incredible Natalie Puche. It doesn't matter what we throw at you—you always find a way to make it work. You're invaluable to us in so many ways; we are blessed to have you in our lives and thank you for always making our visions come alive.

Note to Readers

The anecdotes in this book are used to illustrate common issues and problems that we have encountered, and do not necessarily portray specific people or situations. No real names have been used. This book is comprised of the opinions and ideas of its authors and is meant solely for general informational and entertainment purposes on the subjects addressed in the book. The ideas and concepts in this book are not intended to diagnose, treat, cure, or prevent any medical, health, mental, physical, psychological, or psychiatric problem or condition, nor are they meant to substitute for professional advice of any kind. Specific questions and decisions about treatments should be made in partnership with your health care provider.

Health information changes rapidly. Therefore, some information within this book may be out of date or even possibly inaccurate and/or erroneous. The reader should consult his or her medical, health, psychological, or other competent professional before adopting any of the concepts in this book or drawing inferences from it. The content of this book, by its very nature, is general, whereas each reader's situation is unique. Therefore, as with all books of this nature, the purpose is to provide general information rather than address individual situations, which books by their very nature cannot do.

The author and publisher specifically disclaim all responsibility for, and are not liable for, any liability, loss, or risk, personal or otherwise, which is incurred as a consequence, directly or indirectly, of the use and application of any of the contents of this book.

Any and all product names referenced within this book are trademarks of their respective owners. None of these owners have sponsored, authorized, endorsed, or approved this book in any way. Unless otherwise noted, the authors are in no way affiliated with any brands or products recommended in this book. Always read all information provided by the manufacturers' product labels before using their products. We are not responsible for claims made by product manufacturers. The statements made in this book have not been evaluated by the U.S. Food and Drug Administration.

Introduction: Welcome to the Dubrow Diet

First things first—thank you for picking up this book and for trusting us to guide you through what could be the most profound transformation you've ever experienced. You might think that's an awful lot for a diet book to promise, but this isn't your typical diet book. There are so many reasons why we believe in our program and its ability to change your life. The number one reason is that the dietary principles you will discover in the pages ahead are the very same ones that have helped us transform our bodies and our lives. We live by these philosophies every single day, and not a second goes by without us feeling the benefits of them. (Not to mention how we, ahem, look.) Now, it's your turn.

The Dubrow Diet is a metabolism-targeted plan that focuses on an eating strategy that can help program your body to burn fat and activate the anti-aging ability found in your cells. The combined effect is one that promotes weight loss, boosts energy, and leads to an internal rejuvenation that can improve skin and overall appearance. Talk about a triple threat.

We are thrilled to be bringing the message of this book to you as a couple. We are committed to leading healthy, thriving lives and to helping other people look and feel their best. The fact that we get to share life-changing information with you as a team is a great privilege, and how lucky for you to get two of us for the price of one! You get me: Heather Dubrow, a tried-every-diet, tested-every-product, champagne- and dessert-loving woman, who balances life as a driven entrepreneur, a mom to four kids, and a wife to one of the world's busiest plastic surgeons . . . and did I mention that I need to be ready to appear on camera at a moment's notice? I've worked for years as an actress, a cast member of *The Real Housewives of Orange County*, and a host on multiple shows. No matter what the show, knowing that the scrutiny of an HD camera could be lurking around any corner adds an extra layer of motivation to always stay healthy and on top of my game.

You also get my coauthor and more handsome half, Dr. Terry Dubrow. Board-certified as a plastic surgeon by the American Board of Plastic Surgery, Terry is a graduate of and former fellow at UCLA School of Medicine, where he also served as Chief Resident of General and Plastic Surgery. He has become nationally known—actually internationally known, but I'm trying hard not to brag too much about him!—for his surgical skills and knowledge, partly due to his work on E!'s popular reality show *Botched*. Terry has also published over 30 papers in peer-reviewed surgical journals.

Even though he's a plastic surgeon, Terry's medical expertise goes far beyond what he excels at in the operating room. His knowledge of how the body works, including everything from how our cells and metabolism respond to certain foods to the molecular dynamics that determine how fast we age (or don't age), still blows me away . . . even after 21 years of marriage. He is also insanely dedicated to the study of how we can optimize our biological potential; he regularly pores over the current research to tap into the most advanced ways we can improve our health through diet, exercise, supplements, sleep, you name it.

You might have heard us discuss some of the most cutting-edge ideas on our podcast, *Dr. and Mrs. Guinea Pig*, where we share our insights on just about every health-related topic out there. We've talked about the best form of vitamin D to take, how to deal with your partner's weight gain, why we love beetroot so much, the benefits of CoQ10, how to not gain weight on vacation (while still indulging!), the importance of sleep, and so on. More recently, we've been talking about the Dubrow Diet and how thrilled we are with the results we're seeing in people who have followed the plan. Between the two of us, we've seen a lot of "before and afters"—especially Terry, in his work on E!'s *Botched*—and let me tell you, these are truly profound transformations, inside and out.

But First: The Man (and Woman) in the Mirror

Of course, the very first Dubrow Diet transformations we witnessed were our own. Those were a product of years of research, decades of personal experience, and loads of trial and error. Your journey doesn't have to be nearly as long, complex, or frustrating as ours were. In fact, some of the people who tried the diet before this book lost 40+ pounds in only 10 weeks. And what's even better than the number they see on the scale is that they can't stop talking about how great they feel, how much more energy they have, and how much more engaged they are in their lives.

Both Terry and I have experienced similar benefits by following the principles in this book. He likes to say that sticking to this lifestyle makes him feel superhuman. (If you took one look at his schedule, you'd probably agree with this description). I personally feel great with finally knowing how to eat and live like a human—you know, someone who gets to eat dessert and drink alcohol, eat high volumes of some of my favorite foods, and not spend all day at the gym—while simultaneously feeling better than I've ever felt in my life.

I can only appreciate feeling this way now because I've been in a place where I didn't feel so hot in terms of my weight, energy, and fitness commitment. Terry has had his ups and downs, too . . . and I mean that literally, as he was a yo-yo dieter for a very long time. While this isn't a dietary tell-all, we did want to share with you a little of our dieting histories so you can get a sense of the background and perspectives we bring to this book. We didn't create this diet on paper but instead tested it out in the busy, chaotic lab of our lives over the years, and it took tossing out so many ideas that didn't work before we could arrive where we are today—here, hoping to help you create the best version of yourself.

"You've Expanded Like a Balloon—I Just Want to Pop You!"

I grew up in New York and went to college upstate at Syracuse University. After nearly two decades of living at home and eating what was provided to me, the freedom of college led to a full-on food frenzy. I was in a sorority and, looking back, it seems like most of our time was spent coming up with creative ways to eat. I was obsessed with butter spray—so much so that when we made popcorn, my sorority sisters and I would sit on the kitchen counter and spray every single layer of the popcorn in a giant bowl until the kernels were completely buttered. Almost all my eating had a similar sort of excess involved. I fell in love with the toasted honey buns in the cafeteria and drank beer for the first time, usually alongside some sort of pasta dish coated in cheese. Sound like a typical college life? Well, maybe so, but I went overboard and ate like this almost *every* night!

You've heard about how some people put on the "freshman 15"? In my case, after only five months of college, I had put on almost 30 pounds! When I went home for Thanksgiving, my mom said, "Heather, what's happened to you?! You've expanded like a balloon—I just want to pop you and get the old you back!" It's true; I was so bloated and round I didn't even recognize myself, but it would be another two years before I was ready to make a change.

This started what was to be a long and crazy dieting journey. While still in college, I ended up in the Miss America pageant system, and that's when things really went haywire. I became like a serial dater, except it was with diets instead of guys. This pattern continued through most of my twenties and early thirties. I tried Weight Watchers, Nutrisystem, Jenny Craig, Lindora, the Scarsdale Diet, the Beverly Hills Diet, the Cabbage Soup Diet. And more recently, I've tried the Dukan Diet and the Keto Diet. If there is a diet out there, I've tried it.

Most of these diets had something about them that worked, but none of them provided me with a way of eating that could become part of my lifestyle for the long haul. You know why? Because they just weren't sustainable. Some of them had unrealistic restrictions, such as telling you that you could never eat out again. Others just had food that tasted awful—no thank you, dehydrated food. I remember once taking my dehydrated hamburger to a restaurant and asking for hot water and pouring it over the burger. That is no way to live your life, and for me, once I became a mom, that certainly wasn't going to be the type of eating example I was going to set for my kids.

Looking back, I think a lot of my ideas about food formed at a young age. When I was in college, I met my dear friend Jill. Her mom was really into fitness and healthy eating in a normal, non-obsessive way. When we got ice cream, Jill would get a single scoop on a cone to my three scoops in a cup, slathered in toppings. She would eat pasta and cheese and whatever everyone else was eating; she was never missing out. She just understood how to eat in a way that I didn't. I had never learned moderation or been given a clear sense of healthful foods vs. not-so-healthy foods.

I've seen so many people around me, including family members, struggling with a similar lack of knowledge and the consequential search for the right way to eat. I've crash dieted, I've gotten "skinny fat"—when you look thin but are actually just soft and saggy with no muscle tone because you don't exercise—and several times, I've restricted my calories to the point where I had practically no energy and little excitement about what was happening in my life. It doesn't matter if you're thin when you have no ability to wake up feeling great and make the most of your precious time on this planet.

During this time, I also had little appreciation for the role exercise needed to have in helping me get the body I wanted—and, quite frankly, the body I needed so I could be around for my four kids for as long as possible. Growing up, I wasn't the athlete in the family (that was my sister). I was the actress and singer, so I wasn't naturally pulled into sports. I didn't even know if I was athletic or competitive in that way because I was never put in the position to find out. But let me tell you something I finally realized at the age of 35 with Terry's help: I *do* have an athlete inside of me, and she loves to compete! This was a huge revelation for me. While I'm not so much interested in competing against others (in the gym, at least), I am a fierce competitor against myself, and this is enough to get me out of bed, into my workout clothes, and out the door to hit the weights and the treadmill at least five days a week. (Yes, I just said a minimum of five. More on that in chapter 9, but suffice it to say for now that I love it—and you may, too.)

What this helped me discover is that everyone has some kind of athlete inside of them, and learning to tap into this part of you is one of the keys to feeling young, strong, and energized and to looking amazing as you age. Don't worry: we'll help you uncover the athlete in you no matter how far he or she may be hiding.

After all the years of testing and trying it all, it has finally clicked for me. I'm in a place where I am in control of metabolism and my appetite, where I'm as fit as I've ever been, and I have even more energy than I did 15 years ago—and this is after having four kids during that time. I enjoy eating, I can jump into any activity with Terry and the kids (Max and Nicky are 14, Katarina is 11, and Coco is 7), and I can walk into my closet and feel good wearing anything I want, whether it's a pair of leather jeans and a sleeveless top for dinner, an open-back fitted gown for a red-carpet event, or just leggings and a zip-up for a coffee catch-up with a friend. I'm even guilty of trying on my wedding dress from time to time. (Who doesn't want to be reminded that they can still fit into something from 21 years ago?!)

I want you to think of this book as an invitation to join me in this healthy, energy-infused, happy-with-your-weight place. After so many years, I never thought I'd be where I am today, but I can say it's definitely a better place to be. Especially because Terry is here with me, too. But I'll let him tell you about his path—which has its own distinct twists and turns—because of course it's his story to tell.

My Path to a Perfect Diet

Well, now that Heather finally gave me a chance to write something (love you, honey!), I also want to welcome you to the Dubrow Diet. This is a book we've been dreaming of writing for a couple years now, especially after we had so much fun writing our first book, *Dr. and Mrs. Guinea Pig Present the Only Guide You'll Ever Need to the Best Anti-Aging Treatments*. This book is a natural extension of the first one, with one fundamental distinction—while that book focused primarily on external anti-aging treatments, whether topical or surgical, this book will emphasize ways that you can create an ageless *internal* environment, thereby promoting a more youthful external appearance. In other words, this is an inside job . . . with outside results.

As a doctor, my goals have always been to use my education, training, and experience to help people achieve health and wellness. As a plastic surgeon, my goals are to use my surgical skills to allow people to look and ultimately feel their best. For years, I have seen people try to improve their physical form through surgical procedures like liposuction and various body tucks, when in reality all that was needed was an effective diet and exercise regimen to more safely and effectively achieve their goals. What's so incredibly exciting is that our understanding of how to lose weight rapidly and effectively has progressed radically thanks to new insight into how the body functions to regulate fat stores and insulin physiologically. We now understand key techniques that will allow us to biohack our bodies to lose weight quickly and safely and maintain health and wellness easily over the long term. The Dubrow Diet is built upon many of these cutting-edge developments, which is why I'm so thrilled to be able to share it with you.

In our program, you'll learn how to eat and exercise in ways that will initiate metabolic and molecular makeovers, helping you to not just lose weight but also look and feel younger. Given my medical background, I've always been skeptical of these kinds of promises, even though I know we have a certain degree of control over our biology. However, recent advances in the science of dieting and aging have convinced me that we have more power than I ever thought possible over the hormones that regulate weight and the molecular factors that determine how we age. To put it another way—this is a *very* exciting time to be alive, and I am thrilled to have the opportunity to partner with you to help you look and feel your best.

There's another reason why I'm not skeptical in this case—this diet is drawn directly from the one Heather and I have used in our own lives, so I've seen the results in the mirror and felt the improvements across most areas of my life. I've seen parts of my body that I've worked on for *decades* finally be stripped of stubborn fat. I've also seen my wife (who, as far as I'm concerned, has always been hot) lose pregnancy weight that can be tough to trim naturally in your forties and gain so much energy that she manages to shuttle around four kids; host *Heather Dubrow's World*, one of the top-rated female podcasts in the country, and cohost another with me; and run our skincare line, Consult Beaute. She may not call herself superhuman, but I certainly see her that way.

I consider myself a scientist, which means that I seek understanding at a level that most people don't. This isn't to brag; in fact, this quality of mine is one that often causes Heather to roll her eyes at me or feign falling asleep . . . or to actually fall asleep (it turns out that reading her my studies published in surgical journals works an awful lot like an Ambien). I mention my scientific side because it's a significant player in my relationship with diet and exercise, and it's frankly part of what made me prone to becoming a yo-yo dieter. It's not because I fell prey to the latest dieting fad or whatever diet book was on the best-seller list; it's because science in these areas is always shifting, so when the research is your anchor, it can sometimes be hard to find a steady course.

I've never stopped paying attention to the science of eating, which is really the science of metabolism, which in turn is the science of chemistry, one that revolves around the way our bodies transform units of energy known as calories. There was a time when I believed, as most people did, that achieving your ideal weight was all about "calories in/calories out"—if you burned more calories than you ingested, you lost weight.

In my twenties, I went all in on this theory by pairing intense low-calorie eating with extreme exercising. Though it worked on my body, it didn't work for my life—it was overly restrictive and left little room for enjoyment, making it unsustainable over the long term.

I had learned all about extreme dieting growing up. I was raised by a single mom who was willing to try just about anything that promised dramatic weight loss in a short period of time. I watched as she tried things like liquid diets, Dexatrim, Medifast, and Optifast. And I witnessed her weight go up and down repeatedly over the years. These, too, were just not sustainable; not for her and not for most people. "Crash" diets such as these are also not particularly healthy, and they've repeatedly been shown not to work in the long term.

When I was around 24, I tested the calories-in/calories-out theory another way. I was nearly 20 pounds overweight at the time, so I decided that I would start training for the Los Angeles Marathon. Eventually, I was running between 35 to 45 miles a week. Since I was working out so hard and burning so many calories, I rationalized not just eating more, but also eating plenty of carbs because it was all about carb loading in those days. I was certain that no matter what I ate, I was burning more calories than I was eating, so I would no doubt lose weight.

When I was ready to run the marathon three months later, I weighed myself and was shocked—I had gained a pound. I couldn't believe it. By that point, I was well into my fellowship at UCLA School of Medicine and had developed a detailed understanding of human biology and biochemistry, and yet here I was unable to master my own metabolism. It became clear to me that there was something flawed about the calories-in/calories-out theory, and I ultimately learned what it was: that the type of calorie matters. (There's a metabolic explanation for this, which I'll share with you in chapter 4.)

By the time I met Heather, I was on a pretty strict regimen of chicken and broccoli, no alcohol, no dessert. It's surprising she even liked me considering this was how I lived, but it wasn't long before she made it abundantly clear that this wasn't how *we* were going to live. She's said that she remembers thinking then: *This is not going to work if he doesn't eat dessert.* So, she started converting me and expanding the menu a bit to include things like desserts, red meat, and wine.

A year before we got married, I told her that I was going to lose 20 pounds before our wedding. I wanted to look sharp, fit, and good enough to stand by my stunning bride's side. I spent the year eating more salad and chicken than ever before and exercising constantly. Then, on the day we got married, I said to her: "I'm so close . . . I'm only 22 pounds away." We laughed hysterically at this then, and we still find it funny now, even though it reflects an experience that most of us can agree is pretty frustrating. (It wasn't until later that I discovered that *when* you eat really makes all the difference when it comes to metabolism, but we'll get to more on that.) What this and my previous experiences tell you is that we all have our dieting stories. Despite achievement and accolades and success in other areas of our lives, most of us will hit that insurmountable wall of weight loss at some point, probably over and over again.

So here I was, spending decades trying different dieting and exercise strategies, all the while watching my weight yo-yo up and down, and yet I kept coming up short of my goals. That was until I discovered new developments in the understanding of how the body responds to food and energy consumption. Over the years, I never stopped scanning the science of nutrition, and it finally paid off, revealing a precise way to eat and exercise that has programmed my body to burn fat and drop weight rapidly in a safe and sustainable way.

By following the program in this book, I have, for the first time in my life, created exactly the body I want, and I've been able to sustain it for years. Now what I want is for you to be able to say the same. Our diet plan is also based on anti-aging science that recently won the Nobel Prize. You will learn how to eat in a way that—if you adhere to it properly—can help you turn back the clock on aging, initiating an internal rejuvenation that will increase your energy and reveal itself not just on the scale but in the mirror, too, where you'll see better, younger-looking skin. Of course, under that skin, your internal organs will also be thanking you because they will be operating optimally, setting you up for a longer, healthier life.

How to Fix a Botched Metabolism

When it comes down to it, weight gain and weight loss are matters of metabolism, which is the process by which your body converts what you eat and drink into energy. To create change, then, we must gain control over our own metabolism. This includes developing an understanding of how certain foods trigger certain hormones, (e.g., sugary, starchy foods stimulate the hormone insulin) and discovering metabolic secrets—the biggest revelation of all being that *when* you eat might be even more important than what you eat when it comes to your weight. This is a secret that many who are tapped into more under-the-radar weight-loss trends have known for years. It's a secret that is supported by cutting-edge dietary science, which we're going to expand upon in chapter 1.

Here are some of the benefits you'll experience when you start to follow the plan outlined in this book. In *The Dubrow Diet*, you will learn how to eat in a way that can help:

- Produce fast, safe weight loss by reprogramming your cells to go after stored fat for fuel
- Lower insulin and normalize blood sugar through the use of meal timing and selective food choices
- Fight off inflammation, specifically the type that is linked to inflammatory disorders such as atherosclerosis (the hardening and the narrowing of the arteries due to plaque), type 2 diabetes, and Alzheimer's disease
- Enhance mitochondrial health by increasing DNA repair and activating a process known as autophagy, your cells' self-cleaning process and an anti-aging rock star

Ideally, the metabolic correction you inspire by changing the way you eat will have a collective effect, improving not just your health and longevity but also producing noticeable changes in matters unrelated to weight. So much of your daily experience is defined by your metabolism, including your energy levels, mood, and clarity of mind. When you recognize and take hold of your power to control your metabolism, you can truly change your life. Consider the pages ahead a handbook on how to create this metabolic control. Here's what's to come in the book:

In part 1 of *The Dubrow Diet*, you'll learn all about the core principle of the program, the importance of reestablishing a connection with your appetite and how this plan will help you with that, and the process of autophagy and its impressive anti-aging effect.

Part 2 is all about the phases of the diet. In the first four chapters in this section, you'll discover all the diet details you need to know, a survival guide to help you get started and stay on track, and food lists and meal planners.

(There are recipes, too, created from the food lists and featured in the meal planners, which you'll find in the back of the book starting on page 143.) We'll also share a sample day from our own lives so you can see how the Dubrows make the Dubrow Diet happen. In chapter 8, you'll learn how to make your commitment to healthy living stick. This includes taking a look at the influences in your life and connecting with the many incentives to take care of your body, especially as you age.

In part 3, we'll introduce you to the essential Dubrow Diet "accessories"—exercise and supplemental support—followed by some of our favorite recipes. These will all prove invaluable to you as tools you can use to boost your success on the plan. Exercise is especially important, as its role in establishing robust health and greater metabolic control cannot be underestimated. We've found a specific exercise practice that is efficient, fat-burning, strengthening, supported by science, *and* customizable. You'll read all about it in chapter 9.

Now that you know what's ahead, we're sure you're ready to dive right into *The Dubrow Diet*. Thanks for trusting us to guide you through this transformation, and we cannot wait to hear about your results!

Part One

The Secret and the Science

Chapter 1

What the F***?!

"What the . . . *Fast*?! No way."

That was my first reaction to Terry's big diet secret that he shared with me one night a few years ago. He had been experimenting with his weight practically every day since I'd met him and had pretty much always been disappointed with the results. His stubborn stomach fat drove him nuts (I think this is one of the few things that all men and women can relate to!), and he wanted to feel leaner, stronger, and younger. With an increasingly demanding surgery and TV schedule and our crazy busy kids, there was no room for slowing down.

At the time, I had noticed that his body was changing. He seemed to be leaner in ways I had never seen before. He was more pumped up about life than usual—and that's saying a lot because he is usually pretty darn pumped up. And so I asked him, "What'cha been doing, honey? You look great."

"I'm fasting," he said. "I feel *amazing*, like superhuman amazing. My body is a fat-burning machine. My brain is crisp and clear. I have never felt better in my life."

Now, when someone who is almost 60, a plastic surgeon, and a chronic dieter says that, you pay attention. What I mean is, this is someone who has direct access to the cutting edge of everything; he's obsessed with the science of weight loss (which he refers to as a matter of metabolic mastery) and anti-aging, and he's a constant seeker of answers to the question of how we become the best version of ourselves. If he was onto something, it had to be out-of-this-world good.

Of course, like most people, I sort of shuddered when he said the word "fasting," but I asked him to tell me more. Terry told me that his last meal of the day was the dinner we always had together, always with some wine or cocktails, maybe sake. In the morning, he would just have coffee, and then around one o'clock he would grab a nice, big, satisfying lunch. Dinner was again later in the evening, usually a meal of a high-quality lean protein, like salmon, and a variety of vegetables. It sounded so simple.

Once he started talking about this new eating schedule, he couldn't stop. The research was "mind blowing" . . . his energy was "off the charts" . . . his body "shredded." When someone is this enthusiastic, you can't help but get excited, too—and want to join in.

The Accidental Faster

The funny thing is when I really started looking at when I was eating, it was very similar to Terry's schedule. I had a different process in the morning, but the first hours of the day never involved a big meal. I was typically too busy shuttling the kids around, getting in a workout, and then heading off to Los Angeles to record a podcast or meet with producers. My schedule, it seemed, had turned me into an accidental faster.

I used to be really into eating a bagel first thing in the morning, but it made me feel bloated and tired, and my body seemed to be stuck at soft and squishy in all the wrong places . . . butt, belly, thighs. You know the spots I'm talking about. Those "trouble zones," as magazines like to call them, like they're places we're supposed to avoid. Hello, they are on our bodies, so we can't just get away from them!

The bagel bloat also interfered with my workouts, which I was becoming increasingly infatuated with. (We'll teach you how to discover your inner athlete on page 127.) Working out *before* eating, on the other hand, made me feel slim, strong, and unstoppable, and it turns out this wasn't just in my head—there's a ton of research, which you'll read about in chapter 9, that shows exercising in a "fasted state" is a proven way to supercharge fat burning.

When I started paying closer attention to my eating schedule and making it consistent, I began to get the same sort of life buzz that Terry was experiencing. My whole body seemed to tighten; I just loved how I felt, whether in a bikini, in a glamorous gown on the red carpet—I even felt good naked. Part of this was because my skin also appeared tighter and seemed brighter. And, while I had never been a slacker parent, I noticed that I had become an even better one—I was excited about doing activities (even athletic ones!) with the kids, mostly because I had the energy to do them.

So, it turned out that Terry really was onto something, something that, as my kids would say, is *everything.* In *The Dubrow Diet,* we have taken this "everything" and turned it into a comprehensive eating and lifestyle program that you, too, can follow. At the core of the program is an eating schedule, what we call *interval eating,* that has helped us finally, after decades of being unsuccessful dieters, go from skinny fat and chubby fit to our healthy, ageless bodies.

I think you'll be amazed to discover that changing your schedule is easier than changing your diet. (This isn't to say there won't be essential changes made to *what* you're eating, but the focus is modifying *when* you're eating.) Interval eating isn't just a fad; in fact it's based on a practice known as intermittent fasting that people have followed for hundreds of years, and there is strong science supporting its efficacy when it comes to burning fat from your body. I don't want to steal Terry's thunder, though, so I'll let him fill you in more on what exactly interval eating is, how it works, and why you'll want to start following it today.

Interval Eating: An Introduction

When I was a general surgery resident at UCLA Medical Center, I had to work incredibly long shifts. I'm talking 48 hours straight, home for 8 hours, and then back for another 48. You're in the operating room a lot of the time, often performing surgery on trauma patients who have come in through the ER. In other words, this is not like normal life where you can eat, sleep, and hang out whenever you feel like it.

What was interesting about this time in my life—well, there was a lot that was interesting about it, but I'll save those juicy stories for another book—was how my weight responded to this schedule, and the way that I had to eat because of it. Out of necessity, I would go extended periods of time without eating and then eat as much as I could when I had a break. I remember a three-month-long period in trauma surgery where I would eat nothing for 16 hours and then eat anything I wanted during an 8-hour window. And I lost weight! I felt alert and energized, capable of pushing through the long, demanding hours and the intense, high-pressure work that frequently involved performing lifesaving surgeries.

This was my first introduction to what we would clinically call fasting and feeding cycles, or intermittent fasting, or what Heather and I have come to refer to as interval eating. Now, it wasn't as though I had stumbled upon some unknown dieting discovery—taking an extended break from eating was at the time scientifically known to have not just metabolic benefits but healing ones as well. This is part of the reason why patients are required to fast before many types of surgery—the primary reason is to prevent aspiration of food and drink into the lungs, but secondarily, fasting has powerful effects on postoperative recovery. When important regenerative resources, such as oxygen-rich blood, don't have to be tied up with digestive processes, they can be sent directly to the surgical site to initiate immediate healing. It also appeared to help me recover from years of yo-yo dieting.

It wasn't until years later that I would return to this idea of on-off eating cycles. Because the practice had initially entered my life as essentially a job requirement, I didn't isolate it back then as a strategy to maintain my ideal weight. What brought it back into the picture for me was the phenomenal science, the irrefutable evidence that proved taking regularly scheduled breaks from consuming food was perhaps the ultimate way to control body weight, not just because of one effect, but a combination of effects. Here are a few of the standouts:

- **Reliable weight loss.** Researchers at the University of Illinois at Chicago found that what's referred to as intermittent fasting can lead to reliable, sustained weight loss—over a pound per week. Our own test group revealed that combining this eating schedule with a greater intake of specific foods increased the weekly weight loss to 1.8 pounds per week.
- **Targeted weight loss.** Better yet, some of the weight loss in this study and in other studies done on intermittent fasting was shown to occur specifically in the abdominal region. This is good news for your bikini body and for your health, as belly fat, especially the deep belly fat known as visceral fat, is particularly unhealthy. Visceral fat wraps itself around vital abdominal organs, such as the stomach and liver, and can prevent them from doing their jobs properly. Visceral fat also increases your risk for type 2 diabetes and heart disease and has been linked to breast cancer in women.
- **Sustained weight loss.** A leading researcher in the field of "human appetite control" in the United Kingdom compared groups of people who followed a fasting diet, a very low-calorie diet, and a low-calorie diet. She found that people in the first group lost the most weight, and—this is huge—they maintained most of their weight loss at the one-year mark. The calorie restrictors (both groups) did not fare so well; most participants had regained weight. As a former yo-yo dieter, I can vouch for the long-term effects of intermittent fasting—I've never maintained my weight and fitness for as long as I have eating this way. It's been five years now and I've never gone up more than five pounds.

I don't know about you, but all this science-backed evidence hits all my checkboxes for a dream diet, mostly because it promises to give me exactly what I want. And I love getting what I want.

What's fascinating is that these benefits come from adjusting when you eat and not as much what or how much you eat. (We have found that certain foods do help improve results, and we will encourage you to eat selective, quality foods, but at its core this is not a calorie-monitoring diet.) Your physiology—that is, how your internal mechanisms work to keep your body running—appears to operate at its best when activities are done at intervals. It's a principle that holds true not only when it comes to eating but also with exercise, where high-intensity interval training (HIIT) has proven to be wildly effective. (In fact it's so effective, I like to refer to it as the plastic surgery of exercise because it sculpts like no other. More on this in chapter 9.)

HIIT, which you've probably seen promoted all over the place, operates on a schedule. The schedule typically has you go from exercising hard to recovering, or from a "work" period to a "rest" period. Heather and I have applied this very concept to the practice of eating, but the "working" period is going to be way more fun because you don't have to break a sweat, unless you're eating something spicy. As an interval eater, you will learn how to rotate between periods of refueling and resetting. The reset happens in your metabolism, which is where a major adjustment needs to take place if your goal is to lose weight. Your average day will then look like this: reset, refuel, and then reset. Seem simple? Well, that's because it is, and the results are incredible.

What's not so simple is what happens internally with your metabolism. Metabolism is inherently complex because there are many players involved in converting what you eat and drink into energy. The easiest way to describe what happens to your metabolism when you become an interval eater is to say that you become a fat burner. Your cells will literally start to seek out stored fat to use as fuel. To understand the significance of this, it helps to know a little about how your metabolism works.

Nice to Meet You, Metabolic Miracle Worker

Eating is essentially a process by which energy changes form or is converted. Just like your car "digests" fuel and converts it so it can power the engine, your body digests food and converts it so that the trillions of reactions occurring within can conduct themselves. But the body doesn't see food as one uniform fuel; it sees different parts referred to as macronutrients, categorized as carbs, fats, and proteins. Each of these is responded to and utilized in a different way.

The hormone in charge of this response and utilization is insulin. One way to think of insulin is as a sort of macronutrient chauffeur. It takes carbohydrates, which quickly become glucose, and drives them straight to your cells, where it is used for energy. When you eat foods containing protein, insulin will also be released by the pancreas, although to a lesser degree. Most proteins will get broken down into amino acids, but some may be converted to glucose.

Fats are the only macronutrient that don't stimulate insulin and they have to find their own way, but don't worry about their fate—they'll manage to get absorbed or used as a slow-burning fuel source.

Most of the time, we ingest more food than our bodies can use at one time. Insulin helps again here by linking any leftover glucose molecules together to form glycogen, which is stored in the liver. Once the liver is at capacity, any additional glycogen is converted to fat and stored away in various parts of the body, including the thighs, belly, and buttocks.

The trouble with this stored fat is it is relegated to third in line as an energy source. Because the body is naturally efficient, it will always go for the glucose and the glycogen first since they are easier to convert to energy. Last on the list is your stored fat. When we eat consistently and constantly, we offer up a continual supply of glucose and glycogen, which pretty much says to our stored fat, "Please stay with me. *Forever.*"

The solution? You have to give your metabolism a reset period. You create this reset when you become an interval eater and learn to take a break from eating. By doing this, you make your body work for its fuel. After about 12 hours (the exact time depends upon the individual), it will have burned through glucose and any glycogen found in the liver and various tissue and then head straight for your stored fat to keep the body running without interruption. Buh-bye fat that would otherwise be your lifelong companion!

How to Become an Interval Eater

The key is to ensure that your reset interval is *at least* 12 hours. We have found that the ideal reset interval time is 16 hours. Here's why:

- **It's not that difficult.** You may not believe us now, but after two or so days of interval eating, you'll see it's not as hard as you might think (see the next chapter for why it gets easier).
- **It fits into your schedule.** No one really has time or, for that matter, enjoys the quick bowl of cereal they're cramming into their mouth first thing in the morning, bites taken in between mascara and managing their kid's meltdown. So, why not skip it? Unless you've got the time to start cracking eggs, it's mostly sugar (glucose!) anyway, which means you are simply providing immediate energy rather than programming your body to use fat as fuel.
- **It provides steady, consistent results.** When you follow an interval eating schedule of a 16-hour reset period, then 8-hour eating period, 16-hour reset period, and so on, you ensure reliable, repeated bouts of fat burning.

Now, with that being said, we have created the phases of this diet to ensure that it is sustainable for everyone, including those who may find 16 hours a bit too long and/or those who are OK with slightly slower results. Here's a preview of the phases:

Phase 1: Red-Carpet Ready. This is a two- to five-day metabolic boot camp. It requires full dedication to a 16-hour reset/8-hour refuel schedule. This phase is designed to shock the system and provide an essential appetite adjustment by resetting the satiety center in your brain (i.e., your internal "am I hungry or full" meter).

Phase 2: Summer Is Coming. It's time to reach your goal weight with this phase, which you can customize by selecting the right speed for you:

Slow (average weight loss: .5–1.5 pounds per week)
12-Hour Reset/12-Hour Refuel
Comes with: One magical Cheat Moment (snack, side, or sweet) per week

Medium (average weight loss: 1–2.5 pounds per week)
14-Hour Reset/10-Hour Refuel
Comes with: One gooey, glorious, get-whatever-you-want Cheat Meal per week

Fast (average weight loss: 2–4 pounds per week)
16-Hour Reset/8-Hour Refuel
Comes with: One splendid, splurge-full Cheat Day

Phase 3: Look Hot While Living Like a Human. We all want to maintain our results, but maintenance is for cars—let's continue looking hot instead! During our version of a maintenance phase, you will discover how to practice the principles of this program long term, while also ensuring you enjoy all the indulgences life has to offer.

Your eating schedule will include five days (you pick which ones) of 12-hour reset/12-hour eating and two days a week (we recommend Monday and Thursday) of 16-hour reset/8-hour eating. This phase reflects how we eat now, unless we have an event to prepare for, in which case we jump back to Phase 1 for a few days.

How Interval Eating Can Activate the Ageless Effect and Protect Against Disease

Most of you have probably picked up this book because you want to lose weight, and we'd be the first to understand that motivation. Yet as each of us has reached our goal weight, I think we've both come to understand that we've gained so much more in our lives compared to what we've lost on the scale.

Following an interval eating schedule has helped us prioritize and plan better by clearing out the "calorie clutter," increased our gratitude for food, and improved our relationship with what we put in our bodies each day. This is saying a lot for two people who were chronic dieters for decades. Our hope is that you experience a similar shift when you follow our program.

There are other research-supported benefits, outside of weight loss, that have been linked to the intermittent fasting element of interval eating. Fasting can help:

- Fight off inflammation and autoimmune conditions
- Trigger the production of growth hormone, which is an anti-aging superstar
- Lower heart disease and type 2 diabetes risk factors
- Put the plastic surgeon within to work by stimulating autophagy and enhancing mitochondrial health by increasing DNA repair
- Improve mental clarity by freeing up resources that were previously devoted to digestion the majority of the time
- Increase brain-derived neurotrophic factor, or BDNF, which is important for learning and memory

Collectively, these have the potential to create what we call the ageless effect. The ageless effect has the power to scale back internal signs of aging that have accumulated over time and, in so doing, initiate the restoration of a younger you. This isn't to say that by following our plan you can literally turn back time, although Harvard researchers did find that fasting can lock our cells' energy producers into a "youthful" state, which suggests that we might be able to freeze time internally speaking, at least for a little while. What you can also do is inspire the type of cellular rejuvenation that can give you better skin, more energy, a sharper mind, and reduced disease risk. Much of this rejuvenation takes place thanks to the cellular cleanup process known as autophagy, which is something we'll tell you all about in chapter 3.

And remember, these are the benefits that come alongside the coveted result of sustainable weight loss. This is some powerful stuff. Ready to learn more about it? Let's keep moving!

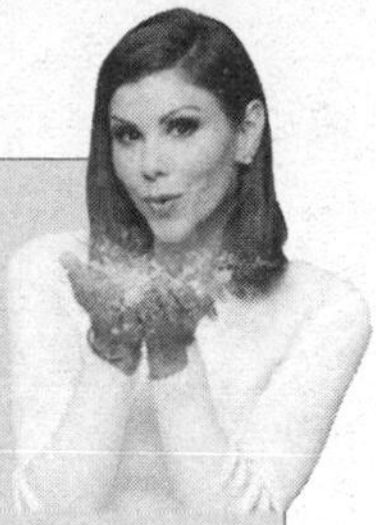

Heather's Hot Corner

So, the cat's out of the bag: you're about to begin a program based on the practice of intermittent fasting. If you're like me, you might think that sounds just a little bit scary. Let me tell you from experience that there's absolutely nothing to be scared of. When you look at it in the simplest sense, all you are doing is skipping breakfast, something you've no doubt done before on a really busy day. In this case, you are skipping breakfast with a purpose: you are pushing back your first meal of the day in order to reset your metabolism and to restore your body to a healthy weight. If you set your mind to it, I have no doubt that this is a change you are capable of making and that you, too, will soon be feeling supercharged in the mornings as your cells shift to burning stored fat as fuel. Get ready for the transformation that lies ahead for you—it's going to be a big one.

Chapter 2

An Essential Appetite Adjustment

We love food just as much as everyone else does. We go to brunch, dig into appetizers, hang around after dinner for dessert and drinks, take our kids for ice cream. But listen: this eating all the time thing has got to stop. You don't need to snack constantly; you don't need small meals every three hours . . . nor do you need to supersize anything ever. Never, ever. (Unless maybe it's a closet. Who doesn't want a super-size closet?!)

When you think about it, the closet is one of the few food-free zones in our lives these days. Pretty much everyone eats in their car or at their desk, in the living room in front of the TV . . . even bedroom snacking is common (which I kind of enjoy, as long as it's during my refuel period!). And once we're out of our houses, forget about it: food is *everywhere.* Just as an experiment, try to spot a place without some kind of snack offering as you go about your day this week. We dare you to find a business without at least a bowl of lollipops on the counter.

What happens when we don't get a break from seeing food is that we are far less likely to take a break from eating food, which can play a vital role in helping reprogram your metabolism. This break is also needed to give your satiety center—the part of your brain that regulates feelings of hunger and fullness, which you might also think of as your appetite satisfaction center—a chance to reset.

A little later in the chapter the satiety center gets more attention, but first a little more on the topic of food availability because this plays an often overlooked role in your relationship with eating and can interfere with your ability to identify true hunger. You may not realize it now but learning to eat out of real hunger, instead of boredom or habit, will be a major part of your success on the Dubrow Diet. Another important shift we'll emphasize is the need to see the food you eat as a source of fuel for the body. This doesn't mean that food can't also be enjoyed, but remembering that the ultimate purpose of eating it is to give your body energy will help you start to make better choices.

Food, Food Everywhere

It's hard to pinpoint exactly when our obsession with food went overboard, but take a look around and you'll see we're in way over our heads: food trucks fill up city streets, malls are dotted with kiosks offering high-calorie coffee drinks and cinnamon rolls, and even hardware stores are in the business of selling candy bars and sodas lest you get famished while shopping for a shovel.

This isn't to complain. Sustenance being available to us on nearly every street corner is a legitimate luxury problem, like stamp it with an "LV" for Louis Vuitton luxury. Yet there's something else that's occurred alongside the rise of food availability: with this luxury problem, we've gained a serious weight problem, one that affects close to three-quarters of the country. The most recent statistics show that more than two out of three people are overweight or obese in America.

This is no small or superficial matter. Too much excess weight is a sign of underlying metabolic mayhem, and if left unattended, it can lead to some serious health concerns. Health risks linked to being overweight or obese include type 2 diabetes, stroke, heart disease, high blood pressure, nonalcoholic fatty liver disease, osteoarthritis, and certain types of cancers.

In Terry's words, this is not the sort of crowd you want to run with . . . but you probably don't need a doctor to tell you that. Most of us have seen one or more of these conditions or diseases disrupt or destroy the lives of people we know and love, or we've experienced the symptoms and side effects of them firsthand.

Of course, food availability isn't solely to blame for the rise in weight gain and obesity, but it certainly hasn't helped matters. For now, just think of it as something that you'll want to open your eyes to as you evaluate your relationship with food and your appetite.

Our Forgotten History: When Food Was Fuel

In recent years, people in the diet world have lost their minds over ancient eating practices. You've no doubt heard about the Paleo Diet, which is based on the idea that eating like our loincloth-wearing ancestors will help us avoid developing so-called diseases of civilization. There are so many diets that have branched off from the original concept of Paleo that it's hard for most people to know what eating like this really entails.

At its core, Paleo is a practice that encourages the elimination of grains, dairy, and legumes (beans, lentils, etc.) and the inclusion of specific fruits, vegetables, and "healthy" fats, such as coconut oil and grass-fed steak. Some have criticized the diet for being too restrictive, even unhealthy, due to too many unsaturated fats in the program.

Say What . . . Carbs Are Paleo?

Published research has suggested that the theory supporting the Paleo Diet is basically a bunch of baloney . . . on white bread. A study titled "The Importance of Dietary Carbohydrate in Human Evolution" (you may have already read about this in *Us Weekly*) found that the original Paleo people ate starches in the form of bark and tubers, which are nutrient- and carbohydrate-rich roots, such as potatoes. The researchers claim that these types of digestible carbs weren't just responsible for filling the bellies of early humans; they also helped fuel their growing brains and accelerated their move toward planetary dominance.

This isn't to scare you away from eating like a caveman or woman, if that's your thing. What's positive about Paleo is the fact that it emphasizes eating foods free of processing and preservatives, a.k.a. "clean" foods. If you've incorporated some of these dietary practices into your life and you like them, keep them.

But we think there's something even more valuable that can be taken away from these prehistoric people than what was on the menu—and that is how they thrived upon the idea of food as fuel. This is one ancient idea that deserves a spot at the head of the modern food table.

The goal here is to step back for a second and consider how you see food; that is, to think about what your relationship is to it. Do you see it as an enemy that you must conquer before you can overcome your struggles with weight? Do you see it as a companion when you're feeling bored or blue, or even when you're just chilling on the couch watching TV (viewing *Botched*, of course!)? Or do you just simply love to eat?

In other words, do you see food as something you fight with, or that serves as a filler or a constant companion with whom you might spend a little too much time? Or maybe a little bit of each of these? There's no right or wrong answer; what's important is that you think about it because if your relationship with food is unhealthy, there's no way you can reclaim your health or reach your ideal weight.

For us, even though we are very different people, we can both say that redefining our relationship with food was absolutely critical to breaking free from the cycle of yo-yo dieting. And this is where thinking back to the Paleo people can be helpful, as their relationship to food was quite different from our modern one.

Ancient people ate food as fuel, according to their journals. (Well, *actual* journals have yet to be discovered, but we know that grocery stores and fast-food drive-thrus weren't around back then . . . so it's safe to assume these people had to do some work to get a meal.) They sought and savored food as a source of energy, a source of survival. They went days without food, fasting, and then feasting upon meals. These people, our biological ancestors, knew nothing of diabetes or obesity; no muffin tops or love handles being complained about then, that's for sure.

You Were Made for Interval Eating

The point is this—our bodies do not have any biological rule or history that says "must have food every two to three hours." Nor do they require any set pattern or time of intake. You know where the concept of three meals a day—i.e., breakfast, lunch, and dinner—came from? *We made it up.* Just like Taco Bell recently made up the idea of a "fourth meal" (no comment on that one). In other words, three meals a day is a cultural, not a biological, construct. Even the idea of breakfast being the most important meal of the day has been exaggerated a bit. Many of the studies supporting this notion were funded by some major players in the breakfast food industry, companies that clearly stood to benefit by breakfast being promoted as essential to good health. In fact, some research has shown that skipping breakfast can reduce your overall daily caloric intake, a win if you're interested in weight loss and proof that waiting to eat doesn't translate to overeating the rest of the day.

As you may recall from the first chapter, the consistent and practically constant consumption of food all but ensures that you will never burn any stored fat from your body. There's simply no incentive for the body to work harder than it must to keep things running; it will always choose glucose from the foods you eat first, stored glycogen from the liver second, and stored fat last.

When you begin to practice interval eating and you stretch the reset interval beyond just a few hours, you will be making the body work for its fuel. And there's an awesome bonus benefit to encouraging your metabolism to get up off the couch—you get an unexpected burst of energy. This energy comes from the adrenaline that is released by the adrenal glands to fuel the cells' quest for food. All of a sudden, you'll notice that you feel like the most focused, driven version of yourself (who may also have an occasional hunger pang to ride out). Do you recall ever feeling this way after eating a big meal? Nope. Because that's just not how your metabolism works.

If you think back to our Paleo pals, this all makes sense. We'd be as done as the dinosaurs if fasting put us into the equivalent of a food coma. When food was scarce, humans needed energy to roam and seek out their next meal, not a nap. There was no food until they hunted it so unless there were leftovers, they had to wait to eat until they could *find* something to eat.

Luckily, most of us don't have to go hunt for our next meal, nor endure the indefinite wait that comes with this need. But we can still benefit from taking a break, and we can do so with the knowledge that our biological makeup has done it so many times before.

Taking Back Control

Don't let this discussion scare you. It's merely meant to encourage you to start paying attention to the forces that drive your eating habits: Do you eat more than you want to because food is always so available? Or because it's part of the eating patterns we've been taught by society?

Only you can answer this question for yourself. You might be surprised to discover that outside forces play a big role in when you eat, how much you eat, and how often you eat. In this book, we're inviting you to be a bit of a rebel against these forces, to retreat from the routine and see what happens when you become an interval eater.

We're sure you're curious about what fasting will feel like, and this again is something that depends a lot on the individual. As much as the processes that control our metabolism are the same, the rate at which they work is determined by several factors, including your age, body weight, height, and sex. This rate is referred to as your basal metabolic rate.

It also depends upon the state of your satiety center (told you we would come back to this). Your satiety center is called the ventromedial nucleus (VMN), and it's located in the hypothalamus, the almond-sized part of your brain that's in charge of maintaining homeostasis, or balance, in the body.

The VMN operates as a sort of appetite command center and can detect changes in fuel stores (energy) through subtle chemical changes in the body. It's the bona fide big boss of your appetite—researchers have said that it "could be the ultimate pathway for control of food intake and obesity." But it also works closely with your stomach, which will respond to hunger or fullness hormones that are triggered by the VMN.

What we really want to take back control of is the communication between the VMN and the stomach. The exchange between these two entities can get locked into overdrive when we eat too frequently and/or too much, and it can "program" you to eat even when you're not hungry. To regain control, we must put the satiety center + stomach conversation into sleep mode so that it can then reboot itself. And this is where your reset interval, or the removal of food for an extended period of time (not just overnight), will come into play.

I wish we could say that the conversation goes quietly down to sleep like a tired toddler. In reality, it's more like trying to get a bunch of teenagers at a sleepover party to go to bed. You might feel a little frustrated as you continue to hear the talking—your grumbling stomach—going on. You might have a desperate moment when you consider snacking until it goes away.

But now that you have the advantage of understanding what's happening internally, you can overcome the urge to eat. You're getting an essential appetite adjustment, and it might finally be exactly what you need to reach your weight-loss goals. The Red-Carpet Ready Survival Guide on pages 58–61 will help provide some tips for getting through the adjustment period.

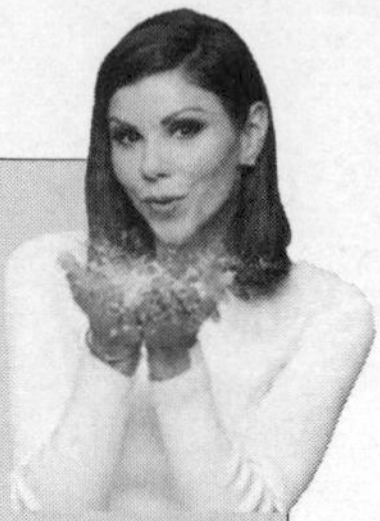

Heather's Hot Corner

Part of your success on this plan will come from a willingness to rethink your relationship with food and your appetite. It's so easy these days to eat out of feelings other than hunger, especially boredom or, on the flip side, busyness and stress. I've definitely caught myself mindlessly making my way through a whole bag of Popchips when reviewing a script or reading work-related emails.

What can we do to break this habit? Wake up! See the snacks and foodstuffs that are everywhere around us for what they are—nutritionally needless temptations. Then, break up with them, at least the processed ones that aren't filling or nutritious. Next, dedicate yourself to creating a fasting discipline that will help you reset your appetite and establish a connection with food as fuel.

Chapter 3

How the Dubrow Diet Activates the Ageless Effect

Since you know that Terry is a plastic surgeon and you've probably assumed that this means we have access to pretty much every youth-restoring surgery, procedure, pill, serum, solution, you name it . . . you might be a little suspect of this chapter, which focuses on the anti-aging benefits of the Dubrow Diet. Why would we use diet and exercise when we don't have to? Is there a little "do as I say, not as I do" going on here?

Not a chance! We're all about the doing of everything you'll find in this book.

Sure, we will rely on Botox occasionally because its wrinkle-relaxing effects are amazing and because TV close-ups are cruel to anyone over the age of 29. And we're both equally obsessed with advancements made in the world of supplements, so we utilize high-quality, concentrated forms of enzymes and nutrients when appropriate. Yet when it comes to going under the knife for cosmetic reasons, neither of us has done that . . . not yet, at least.

Instead, our focus is on living a lifestyle that promotes the type of internal changes that can produce external results. Central to this lifestyle is the practice of interval eating, which research has shown can be a powerful activator of autophagy, an incredible internal renewal process that occurs at the cellular level, where it has the potential to have the most far-reaching benefits.

You might think of autophagy (pronounced aw-tuh-FEY-jee) as a rock star cellular housekeeper, or more specifically like a high-tech Roomba that gobbles up any cellular debris that's naturally created as biological processes occur throughout the body. This is a cleansing process that goes way deeper than any sort of detox or juice cleanse you might try. (Last time I checked, none of those were supported by Nobel Prize–winning science, like autophagy is . . .). Autophagy has been considered key to slowing the aging process and is believed to protect us from developing certain diseases, such as Alzheimer's and cancer.

Since Terry gets supercharged talking about the science stuff, I'll let him tell you more about the awesomeness of autophagy—but be sure check out Heather's Hot Corner at the end for key takeaways!

Awesome Autophagy

Like Heather said, the science around autophagy is convincing, very cool, and cutting edge. As recent as 2016, a Japanese researcher by the name of Yoshinori Ohsumi won the Nobel Prize in Physiology or Medicine for his discoveries about this process involving cellular cleanup. It's definitely something you'll want to know more about if you're interested in flipping on your ageless switch.

To understand how it works, you have to know just a little about what goes on in the body. Here's a quick and hopefully painless rundown.

First off, if you are of the human persuasion, you might want to pause for a second and congratulate yourself—your body is a biological wonder. Being wonderful doesn't come easy; in fact, it takes *a lot* of work. Lucky for us, most of the work occurs involuntarily at the microscopic level, where billions of chemical reactions happen every single second. We're going to focus our attention here on the reactions that occur when energy is created in the body, during the process known as metabolism.

If someone were to describe metabolism to you, you might guess that it was magic. It involves the literal transformation of the food on your plate into energy that fuels your body. That's pretty magical, if you ask me. This transformation includes many steps, and there are countless players involved, including hormones, enzymes, and of course your cells, which is where the energy conversion happens.

Within your cells are tens or hundreds or thousands (depending on the type of cell) of "mini organs" called mitochondria. Mitochondria generate adenosine triphosphate, a.k.a. ATP, a.k.a. your body's mocha java latte. ATP is considered by biologists to be the "energy currency of life"—without it, all your systems would go on strike. Mitochondria also perform the critical function of flagging which cells should be renewed or replicated and which should retire out of circulation.

When ATP is created, by-products known as free radicals are also produced. Free radicals run rampant throughout the body damaging cells, even messing with your mitochondria. An excess of these cellular outcasts can signal trouble and has been linked to weight gain, chronic inflammation, aging, autoimmune disorders, cancer, cardiovascular diseases, and more.

And here, finally, is where autophagy comes into play. The meaning of autophagy is "self-eating"—and while this sounds a little gross, it's exactly what we need to help us out when free radicals have caused damage to cell membranes or mitochondria, or when cellular processes have left any clutter behind. Autophagy is the process that will help gobble up free radicals and a lot of this other cellular debris generated by our internal mechanisms.

A *Facelift for* Your Cells

Autophagy essentially sniffs out any damaged parts or inessential bits and pieces of cells and removes them with surgical precision. I like to think of the process as giving my cells a facelift—and just like a facelift, autophagy aims to remove signs of stress and aging that have emerged over time. What's left behind are rejuvenated cells that are ready to work faster and more efficiently for you.

Unlike a facelift, there's no downtime after you've undergone autophagy, and the only external "side effect" you might notice is brighter, tighter skin. Research has shown that when autophagy declines or is suppressed, collagen production decreases and skin cell turnover slows. These can contribute to increased wrinkles, loss of skin firmness, and thinning skin and leave skin dry, dull, and bland looking. This suggests that if we can stimulate the process, we might soon be seeing some of the benefits staring back at us in the mirror.

The Key to Activating Autophagy

In the first two chapters, we talked about how when you commit to interval eating, specifically the reset interval (when you are fasting), you can help reprogram your metabolism to burn fat and reboot your satiety center to quiet false hunger. This very same reset interval is also what's critical to activating autophagy.

The science says that our internal cellular cleansing process is triggered based on nutrient availability—when there is an absence of nutrients, it is turned on, and when there is an abundance of nutrients, it is shut off. Just like we discussed how taking an extended break from eating can make your body work a little harder for fuel and increase fat burning, so too can it make the body work a little harder at rejuvenating itself.

What's incredible about autophagy is that because it happens on a cellular level, it has the potential to impact your health in several ways. Scientists and specialists in various fields have been studying it recently and producing some encouraging research. Autophagy has been shown to:

- Help control inflammation (possibly by removing free radicals that can accumulate and create an inflammatory state), which is linked to multiple inflammatory diseases, such as inflammatory bowel disease, Alzheimer's disease, and multiple sclerosis
- Provide the building materials needed for the renewal of cellular components (some of the cellular waste products gobbled up by autophagy get recycled into usable "parts")
- Accelerate healing by helping eliminate invading bacteria and viruses that linger after an infection

- Act as "quality control" for your cells by clearing out damaged parts and mitochondria, which can help counter the negative effects of aging
- Enhance metabolic functions by wiping out overworked and over-stressed mitochondria, likely helping prevent the duplication of dysfunctional DNA

Interestingly, when we carry too much weight on our body, the effect of autophagy can be weakened—even more incentive to get started with interval eating as soon as possible! As you work toward programming your body to burn more fat, you'll also be working toward getting the most out of your own internal anti-aging capabilities.

Your #1 Anti-Aging Ally

I truly believe that taking steps to stimulate this internal process is one of the most proactive things we can do to counter the effects of aging. After all, aging is the result of the breakdown and degradation of cells and tissues, and autophagy is one of the few things that can step in and say, "Hey, not so fast." Since autophagy declines with age, we have to strategically work to make it happen and, so far, periodic fasting seems to be the only way to activate it. And now you've got the Dubrow Diet to help you make that happen.

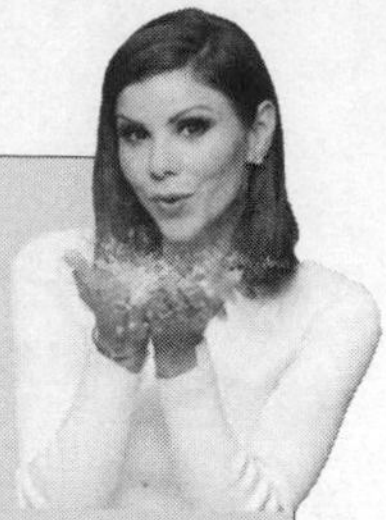

Heather's Hot Corner

Autophagy sounds like something you might find on the menu at a Greek restaurant (makes sense since it's a Greek word!), and if it were, it's definitely something you'd want to order—trust me. When I started consistently following an interval eating regimen, what I noticed was that it wasn't just my weight that changed—my skin seemed tighter and almost started to get a little glow going. Yes, please, to more of all that.

I also love the idea that I'm promoting a spick-and-span internal environment. If you know anything about me, you know I cherish a clutter-free space—and it makes me seriously happy to think about those spotless cells of mine doing good work. Of course, knowing that autophagy can help prevent disease is motivating as well. I love being a mom, and I want to be around as long as possible for my kids!

Part Two

The Phases

Chapter 4

Phase 1: Red-Carpet Ready

We've told you about our long and winding dieting stories, which included a lot of yo-yo dieting for both Terry and me. I want to share with you a little more about my story before we get into the details of the first phase because I think it will help you get into the right mindset to start the Dubrow Diet.

My Journey to Interval Eating

There have been some standout times in my life when I had a lot of weight to lose—after my first year in college, when I had put on more than 30 pounds, and after I had our twins, when I was 60 pounds bigger than normal due to the pregnancy. The rest of the time, I felt as if dieting was sort of like a shadow that I could never shake; it was always with me.

After college, I cycled through every type of diet program you can imagine. My pattern was a little like a country-western dance: "now, take two steps forward, then one step back." This was partly because I often found myself involved in things that required me to be thin, sometimes unhealthily so. I was in the Miss America pageant system for a while, which demanded extreme focus on what I was eating (having to wear a swimsuit onstage can be highly motivating . . . in the short term). I was always trying to learn the specific rules and restrictions of whatever new diet I was about to start.

Later, when I was trying to make it as an actress in Los Angeles, I spent a lot of time drinking Diet Coke, smoking cigarettes, and eating terribly. I remember one time when I was at the most popular sushi restaurant in LA in the '90s; it was *the* spot to be seen and to schmooze, and to enjoy great sushi. You know what I ate? A bowl of raisins . . . with chopsticks. (Thank you, Beverly Hills Diet!) Can you imagine? All this beautiful, nutrient-rich, delicious fish to be eaten, and I'm chewing on wrinkly, sugar-filled dried grapes that had pretty much *nothing* to offer my body. It's no wonder I was skinny fat.

I feel like I spent almost two decades trying to be red-carpet ready. And it was not fun. I've always loved food, but my relationship with it during those years wasn't all that positive. There were plenty of times when I indulged, especially when I would go home to visit my family in upstate New York and my mom would make some of my favorite dishes, and I would just eat and eat, portion control be damned. But those times usually left me feeling crappy, physically and mentally.

Looking back, I can see that there were two major things missing during this time of my life: (1) a focus on eating real, whole foods, and (2) exercise. Like I mentioned earlier, I didn't grow up around people who exercised, and it wasn't something that was encouraged. It's not that it was discouraged either; it's just that some people have families who go hiking or running or even hit the gym together, but that wasn't the way my family was growing up. (I've broken this cycle, as Terry and I are very active with our kids, which is something that makes me incredibly happy.)

Of course, it's only in hindsight that I can see what was missing and what was messed up about my approach to feeling good about my body. I wish someone had taken me by the shoulders when I was younger and said, "Heather, snap out of it! It doesn't have to be this hard."

In a lot of ways, becoming an interval eater is what finally provided the shake-up I needed and broke me out of what I thought was my dieting destiny. I was certain that I faced a frustrating forever of weight gain and loss, of not feeling physically the way I wanted to feel, or of not having the energy I needed to get the most out of my life.

But interval eating helped me jump off that path by giving me a new perspective on food. I've learned to appreciate food as fuel, and I've also discovered that dedicating a smaller window to eating each day encourages me to make better choices about what I put in my body—I go for maximum nutrition, fresh flavors, and strategic indulgences.

I like to think of the way Terry and I feel now as representing a happy ending to our dieting stories . . . or maybe it's the beginning of a new one that will last for the rest of our lives? Either way, we look and feel better than ever. And now it's your turn to create your new beginning as you start the Dubrow Diet.

Think about where your diet story has taken you so far, the ups and downs, and commit yourself to being in control of what happens next—and know that changes are coming. No matter how you look at it, you've got to make changes to your lifestyle if you want to make changes to your body and feel better each day.

Don't act like or even think for a second that you can't do this—make the commitment to change. And remember: though you can't control where you come from or what's happened in the past, you *can* control where you go to—the journey toward the you you've always dreamed of starts now.

Get Red-Carpet Ready

This first phase—what we call Red-Carpet Ready, or RCR—is designed to work as a short and powerful metabolic boot camp; it provides the jolt that your system needs to wake up and start working harder. It can also provide the kind of quick results that have been shown to light a fire under your motivation.

I'm not going to say that you'll see instant weight loss in this first phase, but our early testers of the diet were amazed at how quickly they noticed improvements in how they felt. Both Terry and I have noticed that the first couple days of interval eating make us feel light and lean, and they also introduce a renewed connection to hunger that's essential to establishing a lifelong relationship with healthy eating habits.

We recommend that you follow this phase for at least two days but no more than five. You can select a specific duration based on how much weight you have to lose:

Less than 10 lbs. to lose: 2 days

From 15 to 30 lbs. to lose: 3–5 days

30+ lbs.: 5 days

No matter what your weight-loss goal, after five days you should move into the Summer Is Coming second phase. This is an important point to keep in mind about RCR—this isn't your forever diet. But it is the one we'll begin with because waking up your metabolism is critical to creating the kind of body transformation we want.

What's great about the RCR phase is that you can do it to kick off the diet, but you can also use it later to get yourself back on track, or when you want to look fabulous for an event. We often find ourselves in a position where we have to look good for an event within a short period of time, and we use this phase to get us there. Even if you don't have an actual red-carpet event to prepare for, the Red-Carpet Ready phase will make you feel as though you could make any type of entrance with confidence. It's a truly powerful jump start.

The Big Three: Food Factors That Matter Most

Since we've both followed a lot of different diets throughout our lives, we know how frustrating it can be to try and implement an eating plan that's overly complex or requires you to become a math wizard just to stick to it.

That's why we're leaving calories out of the equation, and percentages, too. Instead we want you to focus on three factors related to food, ideally in this order: (1) when you eat, (2) what you eat, and (3) how much you eat. Yes, it's really no more complicated than that! Here's a little more on what we mean by this.

WHEN. When you eat is of course the key while you're on the Dubrow Diet. You might remember from the first chapter that it takes around 12 hours for your body to burn through its glycogen stores and to start burning fat as fuel.

The Real Deal: What to Expect from a Metabolic Reset

We've established that interval eating is the key to resetting your metabolism. Just to recap, or explain to you for the first time if you jumped right to this part of the book (no judgment—we all do it!), here's what happens when you modify your eating schedule so it includes an extended break from food intake:

- You force your body to tap into stored fat.
- You reset your satiety center, which controls feelings of hunger and fullness (your appetite).
- You activate the effects of the youth-restoring process of autophagy.

The key to tapping into all these benefits is the reset intervals, the length of which will vary in each phase of the Dubrow Diet.

During this first phase, you'll want to follow a 16-hour reset interval, followed by an 8-hour refuel interval. When you stick to this schedule, you give your cells at least four hours to get busy gobbling up stored fat.

WHAT. Next in line of priority is what you're eating; you simply can't leave this out of the equation if you want to create the ageless effect. Although you would probably lose weight in the short term just by following the interval eating schedule, you wouldn't be that happy with your results—a chips and cookies diet does not do your outward appearance or internal environment any favors.

These foods, along with other "standard American diet" favorites, such as French fries, pizza, and soda, can cause premature aging, prolong issues with your weight, result in nutrient deficiencies (which can domino into countless other issues), and lead to the type of metabolic dysfunction that's been linked to diseases such as diabetes, among others.

If you don't pay attention to what you eat, and especially if you eat a diet high in processed foods, you can damage the very same cells that you're trying to rejuvenate with interval eating.

HOW MUCH. Most of us in this country have what I call PDS—Portion Distortion Syndrome. OK, so maybe this isn't an *actual* syndrome, but it does accurately describe our warped sense of how much food we need to eat to satisfy our appetites, and how full our plates need to be when we sit down at home for a meal or have one served to us at a restaurant.

We'll address this further a little later in the chapter, but for now just know that paying attention to how much you're eating can also help recalibrate your metabolism and appetite-related hormones in beneficial ways.

Why You Shouldn't Focus Only on Calories

If you've ever done a calorie-counting diet, you know that it can drive you crazy . . . and consume a lot of time! Who knows what I could've done with the time I have spent looking at nutritional labels on foods—it's at least enough minutes to fill a week of vacation!

As for Terry, you might remember from the introduction that he went through a time where he was obsessed with calories in/calories out—that is, the idea that the only way to lose weight is to make sure that you burn more calories than you consume. He laments that it was mostly unsuccessful for him, but it wasn't until later that he realized why. He can chime in here to tell you more about this revelation . . .

Here's what is flawed about the calories-in/calories-out theory—our bodies don't metabolize all calories the same way. One of the key differences is the degree to which the three different types of calories we consume stimulate the hormone insulin. Each of these calorie types—which you'll recognize by their macronutrient names carbohydrate, protein, and fat—is greeted by a distinct insulin response within the body.

Let me tell you a little about why this matters.

The Importance of Insulin

If you want to put an end to a conversation at a party, just start talking about insulin. Works every time. Even the word itself is a bit of a snooze. But we have to talk about it, at least a little. Here's why: over the years, insulin has proven to be perhaps the most critical factor when it comes to how we store fat.

Insulin is a hormone, which is basically a messenger in chemical form, that is secreted by the pancreas. When you eat food, your blood sugar (glucose) rises, and insulin gets sent out into the bloodstream to get glucose out of the bloodstream and into your cells for use. Like any good messenger, it arrives at its destination—your cells—and knocks on the door, then ushers in glucose molecules to be used as fuel.

Things will continue this way until your cells have received all the energy they need. Any leftover glucose will get stored as glycogen in the liver first and, second, turned into fat through a process referred to as de novo lipogenesis. Your body will then have access to each of these different fuel sources when it's needed, and it will burn through them in the same order they were stored—glycogen first, fat second.

If it sounds complex, that's because it is . . . and I've only scratched the surface, or really just a tiny little speck on the surface of the science of metabolism. But here's the two-second takeaway: when insulin is high, the inevitable result is increased fat storage. And what triggers high insulin? The presence of glucose.

The Dubrow Diet has been designed with these two key factors of fat storage in mind. Here's how you'll keep them in check:

1. By not eating during your reset interval, you will signal a temporary shutdown on the production of insulin, grinding to a halt the genesis of fat.
2. By eating strategically during your refuel interval, you will prevent a glut of glucose from entering the body all at once, thereby keeping insulin levels relatively stable—but never overly high.

The strategy involves paying attention to the macronutrients carbohydrate, protein, and fat and how much you're eating of each. And when I say "how much," I don't necessarily mean that you'll need to keep an eagle eye on food quantities. What you will need to do, however, is develop a sense of dietary direction, one that guides you away from processed carbohydrates and toward vegetables, proteins, and healthy fats.

Meet Your Macronutrients

Chances are when it comes to food, you know your carbs from your fats and your proteins, but you'll do better on this plan if you understand a little of how insulin reacts to each category of calories. Plus, we've dug through some of the best nutrition science to make sure that what you eat first is what will likely be best for your results. Check it out . . .

Carbohydrates stimulate the greatest production of insulin, especially refined carbs such as baked goods and most pastas, breads, and cereals, which contain mostly processed ingredients. We call these factory carbs because that's probably where most of these types of carbs came from. Factory carbs typically provide more glucose than we can use or need at any one time (even if you're running tens of miles a week, as I learned the hard way).

Complex carbohydrates, a.k.a. fresh carbs that are found in vegetables and whole grains, trigger insulin as well, but to a lesser degree. They contain an important fat-burning ally, fiber, which slows the introduction of glucose into the bloodstream. You'll learn more about the importance of fiber on page 86.

When selecting veggies, always go for fresh first. Then, go for green. Deep-green vegetables contain a whole host of benefits. They're rich in folate, magnesium, and antioxidants such as vitamins C, K, and A, which have incredible anti-inflammatory effects. They are also high in thylakoids—tiny compartments found in plants that contain chlorophyll. Chlorophyll allows plants to absorb light from the sun and create energy, and it also has been shown in studies to help reduce body weight.

Researchers studying appetite regulation at Lund University in Sweden tested the effects of certain chlorophyll-rich vegetables and produced some results that could help you adjust to this first phase of the diet (and long term, too, but it will be especially helpful in the early days of interval eating). What they found was that consuming a drink rich in thylakoids—in this case, a mixture of freeze-dried green plant membranes made from baby spinach leaves and a small amount of Swedish blueberry soup—before eating resulted in lower cholesterol levels, significant weight reduction, and a decreased urge for sweets and fats. This reduced craving for sweets and fats is a big deal since ideally it will assist in the reset of your satiety center, or at least make the adjustment a little less uncomfortable.

You can try to replicate the results of this study in real life by eating chlorophyll-rich foods at the start of your meals. This could mean beginning with a green or small seaweed salad or even a smoothie that's loaded with kale or spinach (try our Virgin Piña Colada with Benefits recipe, which contains baby spinach, on page 197). We prefer smoothies to the popular green juices since they retain more fiber and likely a greater amount of the plant membranes we want to consume for their ability to curb cravings. All green vegetables are high in chlorophyll, but green leafy vegetables contain the most. Here are some of the best sources:

- Spinach (the number one source!)
- Arugula
- Lettuce
- Cabbage
- Kale
- Chard
- Collards
- Green beans
- Leeks
- Herbs (cilantro, dill, parsley)
- Seaweed

You'll see a long list of other carbohydrate choices in the Red-Carpet Ready Food List on page 67. But for now, consider this your carb motto: *so fresh and so green will make me so lean*. It sounds silly, but it's true!

When you focus on fresh and green carbs first, you will naturally reduce your overall carbohydrate intake (since you'll already be full), and this is a good thing. It's good because it will help produce some benefits that we think you'll find quite motivating. These include stabilized energy levels, a little more get-up-and-go, reduced cravings, and early weight-loss results, which are key if you're into quick results like me. (I can't help it; I'm a plastic surgeon!) Some of this weight loss will be from water, but this shouldn't matter much—you will still *feel* better as your body composition begins to change.

All that being said, whatever you do, do not try and cut out carbs completely—this isn't a ketogenic diet, which emphasizes strict elimination of carbs and a high intake of fat (see the sidebar for more info on "keto" eating). Carbohydrates can help stimulate leptin, an appetite hormone that makes you feel full.

So that's the skinny on carbs. Next up are proteins, which you'll get from chicken, fish, meat, eggs, dairy, nuts, and beans. Proteins are broken down into amino acids, which are often referred to as the building blocks of the body. This is because they bond together to form your cells and in turn muscle and other tissues. The proteins that you eat will stimulate a minimal insulin response.

Fats, such as those found in oils, nuts, seeds, and all animal products, are the only macronutrients that don't require insulin. They get broken down into fatty acids by enzymes released by the pancreas. These fatty acids then get used by your muscles for energy or stored in your fat cells for later use.

Now, based on the lack of insulin response, you might assume that this diet would be all about eating fat. But some research has shown that eating fat will trigger the brain to produce the compound galanin, known to be an important appetite regulator. Galanin specifically increases the craving for more fat, especially in someone who's overweight and/or obese. (Excess weight is an indicator that there is at least some degree of metabolic dysfunction present.) Galanin can also work against our efforts to lose weight by driving the cells to use carbs (i.e., glucose) for energy instead of fats.

For this reason, we recommend that you not overdo it with fat or high-fat proteins in the first two phases of the diet. It's during this time when your satiety signals are increasing in strength that you are most prone to the craving-causing effects of galanin. The good news is that once your metabolism and appetite centers have been reset, this sort of fat-craving loop doesn't occur, and you can increase your intake of healthy fats from foods such as avocado, olive oil, and nuts and nut oils.

The Veto on Keto

If anyone you know has mentioned being on a "keto diet," what they're referring to is a ketogenic diet. The goal of this diet is to force your body into a metabolic state known as ketosis. In ketosis, your body has shifted entirely from using glucose as fuel to using what are referred to as ketones, which are the by-products created when fat is burned. So, when you are in ketosis, you are in full-blown fat-burning mode. Sounds great so far, right? The catch is that on a ketogenic diet, your diet needs to consist of about 60 to 75 percent fat, which might include doing things like eating tablespoons of high-fat oils to ensure that you've eaten enough fat for the day. For most people, this is not a sustainable way of eating.

In the Dubrow Diet, you will benefit from the part-time ketogenic effect created by intermittent fasting, all while enjoying more liberal food choices. (Not to mention more satisfying. Tablespoons of "high-fat oil"? Yuck!)

Do You Have PDS?

In the introduction, I mentioned Jill, my dear friend since college. I was drawn to Jill when I met her because she was funny and stylish, and because she was just so relaxed when it came to eating. She always ate whatever we were all eating, but never *as much* as the rest of us (she definitely didn't have Portion Distortion Syndrome). She was healthy and she seemed to enjoy the portions of her food.

It probably wasn't just some innate gift that she had—I'm sure her parents guided her in a certain way that other parents didn't. It's silly to think that all these years later I can still remember her seemingly perfect portions, but it was imprinted in my brain for some reason. Maybe it stands out now more than ever because it seems like healthy portions are hard to find these days, and who even knows what a "healthy portion" is anymore?

In the beginning of the chapter, we discussed the big three food factors you should pay attention to on this plan: when, what, and how much. As you may have guessed, we've reached the "how much" part of things. And even though it's last on the list of priorities, it absolutely has to be on your radar if you want to see the best results out of the Dubrow Diet.

We don't want to harp on portions too much because we have both been on diets that were all about portion control, and they usually came with a heaping side of misery, especially those that required foods to be weighed. Our goal instead is for you to become thoughtful about what you eat without overthinking it.

Paying attention to how much you're eating is important because eating too much can continue to overstimulate your appetite center and interfere with your efforts to initiate a reset. It's also important because it's too easy to fall into the trap of just eating what's served to you, especially when you go out to eat, and not even pausing for a moment to consider if it's more than what you actually need. This is one of the reasons why we recommend no eating out for this phase, if you can manage it. Making your own meals will help ensure there are no mystery ingredients and give you a greater connection with and awareness of what—and how much—is going into your body.

We live in a culture, too, where we are constantly susceptible to single-unit splurges. We tend to grab something that's in a single bag, box, or bottle and see it as a one-time, one-person snack. I try to teach our kids about this type of stuff when we're at the movies and they each grab a box of candy or some type of snack. I have them flip over the package and read the serving size. Even if the box of chocolate candies says it only has 210 calories, you've got to read the serving size info for the complete picture. If it says, for example, 2.5, then what you're really looking at is 525 calories in that box. We may not be counting calories on this plan, but even our seven-year-old knows now that this is more candy calories than one person needs as a treat in one sitting.

As you begin the first phase of this diet, start thinking about serving sizes and appetite-appropriate portions. If you pick up a packaged food (which you ideally won't be doing too often on this plan), scan the number of serving sizes as a way to mentally make some adjustments. And when you sit down to enjoy a meal, give what you've eaten a little time to settle before you assume that you're going to need more. You'll be amazed how waiting even five minutes before helping yourself to seconds will give your brain/stomach conversation enough time to let you know, "Actually, I'm fine. I've had enough to eat."

You'll also see serving size recommendations when you take a look at the food list for this phase. There are tons of options of what to eat, along with an indication of how much from each category you should have each day. These aren't hard-and-fast rules, and no one's going to slap your wrist if you take an extra spoonful of zucchini. They are, however, based on early testing of the diet and reflect the general intake that has been shown to produce some of the best body transformations we've ever seen.

Chapter 5

Red-Carpet Ready Survival Guide, Food List, and Meal Planner

Now that you understand the principles of the plan, it's time to put them into practice. If the thought of getting started makes you a little nervous—which I think is totally normal before beginning anything brand new—I recommend that you try and view those nerves not as feelings of anxiety but rather excitement. Now is the time to get excited about resetting your metabolism and making progress toward your goal weight, or to feel pumped about activating autophagy, your body's most powerful anti-aging ally. I want you to get excited about going on this journey with us, in the same way you would if you were about to take a trip to a place you've always wanted to go. In this case, you're heading straight toward your goal weight (hopefully on a one-way ticket)!

1. **Establish your mindset.** It's imperative that you get it set in your mind that you are ready to go and you are ready to make a true commitment to the plan. Push the doubts out of your head, and forget about going only "half in"—you deserve more than that. If it helps you to go all in, keep in mind that this is just a two- to five-day phase. You've got this.

2. **Make a record of your "before" body.** Step on a scale that you'll have access to throughout the program and make note of your current weight. Save the number into your phone's Notes, write it in an email to yourself, or jot it down in a journal. Wherever you put it, just make sure it's somewhere you'll remember when you want to check your progress. If you'd prefer to not use a scale, or you want an additional way to measure success, you can take a photo of yourself in a swimsuit or another revealing outfit.

   No matter which way you choose to record your before body, remember that this is for documentation purposes only. There's no need to tack on any self-judgment or self-defeating statements when you see the number or snap your picture.

   Since this is a relatively short phase, we recommend waiting until you're done with it to check your progress. In the next phase, you'll check in with your body on a weekly basis (if you want to); more details on page 81.

3. **Read the Red-Carpet Ready Survival Guide.** In this guide, we offer you some essential tips and strategies for success. Without further ado, here it is . . .

The Red-Carpet Ready Survival Guide

1. **Don't start fasting on a Monday!** Mondays are rough. Don't make them rougher by adding something new into the mix. We recommend starting on a Wednesday or Thursday.
2. **Don't fear the rumbling.** You can probably tell by now that we don't sugarcoat things much. So, it might not surprise you when we say what other diet book authors won't say to you: at the beginning of this diet, you will feel some hunger. And let's face it, that can suck a little! But this temporary feeling is not something you should fear or feel worried about; in fact, it's a sign that the metabolic adjustment you want and need is taking place.

After it's been about 12 hours since your last meal, your stomach will likely start sending signals that it's time for something to eat. These signals could include a low rumbling, which is the result of muscle contractions in the stomach. This sound is produced after you've eaten as well, but it's muffled by muffins . . . and any other foods you've ingested, making it harder to hear.

Your brain is responsible for triggering all the tummy talk. When your brain senses your lowering glucose levels, it will tell your stomach to release some ghrelin, a hormone known as the hunger hormone. And this will cue the stomach muscles to contract, kicking off the concert from your core.

Ghrelin is both our nemesis and our biggest ally. We've got to be stronger than the feelings it triggers, but knowing it's there is a sure sign that the internal shift we've been working toward is taking place. Yes, it's really happening—your body is stalking your fat cells and ready to burn them for fuel.

3. **Keep a coffee caddy with you at all times.** Caffeine is an anorectic, which means it works as an appetite suppressant. If you feel hungry, sip on some coffee or tea (this does *not* mean a ginormous blended coffee drink or a bottled sweet tea—see page 62 for specifics). My go-to is a Dunkin' Donuts Keurig cup with a little stevia and sugar-free vanilla creamer; it's like a donut in a cup! Caffeine not your thing? Decaf coffee has proven to be even more effective than regular at lessening hunger and increasing levels of PYY, an appetite-suppressing hormone produced by the body. Pick the brew that works best for you, so long as you watch your sugar intake with it.
4. **Check your calendar.** Although we've discovered that it's almost easier to stick to our interval eating schedule on vacation—we sleep in later, which eats up fasting time, and usually get right out of the hotel and into the world for some adventure—you probably shouldn't start the program while you're traveling for work or fun.

Pick a time when you have at least a couple weeks without any major obligations or shifts in your normal schedule. It won't take long for you to get good at eating according to the Dubrow Diet, but it will take a little bit of practice before you feel like an absolute pro.

5. **Fill your calendar.** At the same time, you don't want to just sit around your house waiting for your first meal of the day. Plan to get some kind of physical activity in the morning (maybe even something intense; see chapter 9 on exercise), and then get busy working. Set up a meeting, run errands, sort through the laundry pile . . . and don't even think about opening that refrigerator door unless it's a secret door to where you store your jump rope and some weights and you want to grab them for a quick workout.

6. **Let this be our little BDS** . . . that is, our Big Diet Secret. Of course, we love our friends, and spending time with them is important. But here's a tip that we think will help you immensely, especially in the early days of trying to establish a new eating schedule for yourself: *don't tell your friends what you're doing.*

   Now, this may be opposite of what you've heard before about creating accountability or building a support system around you, but the truth of the matter is if your friends aren't following the same plan as you, they'll probably try to sabotage it. Not because they are bad people but because they are humans who have tribal instincts, and if you aren't doing the same thing as them, they'll start to feel uncomfortable or question your plan of action and the program that's going to get you there.

   So, just be cool and plan accordingly. Don't schedule a get-together at a restaurant during your no-eating interval; either push it until your fasting hours have ended or meet for a workout or walk instead.

7. **Resist the splurge.** When the time comes for you to eat your first meal of the day, don't just go straight for the gorge. You know why? Because you'll feel like crap. You'll go from feeling light,

lean, and energized to full, fatigued, and fat in just a matter of minutes. To avoid overexcited overeating, plan ahead by knowing what you're going to eat for your first meal. Make it quality, and let the feel-good juices start flowing.

8. **Drink a lot of water.** Aim to get around eight glasses of water a day. It's hydrating, filling, and has no calories! Drinking enough water can help maintain healthy circulation and digestion, prevent premature wrinkling, and ensure that your kidneys have plenty of fluid to filter out waste. It should be noted that drinking water is absolutely allowed and encouraged during your fasting window. (See the list of what's allowed on pages 62–63.)
9. **Increase your electrolyte intake.** Electrolytes such as potassium, sodium, magnesium, and calcium can help as you adjust to a lower carbohydrate intake. One good source of these electrolytes is coconut water. Coconut water is especially high in potassium, a mineral that will decrease some as your body burns through stored glycogen (potassium helps metabolize glucose). Just one eight-ounce serving can be helpful, but be sure to get it unflavored and drink it only after you've completed your fast. In other words, just because it has the word "water" in its name doesn't mean it's permissible during your fasting period.
10. **Take helpful supplements.** Add a daily multivitamin, vitamin D, and a beet supplement to help boost energy and support your body during weight loss. It's generally OK to take supplements on a fasted stomach, along with regular medications. However, it's important to always check with your doctor first. If upset stomach occurs, then wait until you've eaten to take anything. See chapter 10 for more on supplements.
11. **Use the food resources we've provided.** The food lists, meal planners, and recipes included in this book are there to help make sure you're never at a loss for what to eat while following the plan. Use them!

The Short List: What You Can Consume While Fasting

You probably noticed that there are certain items that we allow ourselves to have during the fasting period. We limit ourselves to beverages and supplements that have minimal calories and no sugar. Since our primary goal is to ensure that insulin stays low and that we stay in fat-burning mode, the no sugar part of this is key (remember, sugar triggers insulin). Liquids can be helpful in easing hunger, since they will add volume to your stomach and create at least a temporary feeling of fullness. You can drink any of the following during your reset interval, but be sure that the total calories from whatever you add to your coffee plus those in the beet drink and green drink doesn't exceed 100 calories. If you notice that your results or progress change based on any additions you make, don't be afraid to scale back or make adjustments.

- **Water.** I like flat water, but sparkling is good, too. One of my favorite things to do is to put some water in a reusable glass bottle and squeeze a little lemon and lime in there, and then add some fresh mint. Or if I want spicy, I'll add a dash or two of cayenne pepper to the water and lemon juice mix. Then, I'll carry this bottle with me throughout the day and refill as needed. You can add other fruits and herbs, but just don't eat the fruit unless you've reached the end of your fasting interval.

- **Coffee.** Like a lot of people, Terry goes straight for coffee in the morning. I can't drink it first thing because it gives me heart palpitations and is a little too hard on my stomach, so I'll save my coffee for a little later in the day. I generally don't do well with dairy, so I'll add nondairy creamer. Terry does nondairy creamer, too, but I think mostly because he just prefers the taste of it. You can add one to two teaspoons of skim milk or coconut milk to your coffee, if you'd prefer. Feel free to add cinnamon or nutmeg to your coffee as well, but stay away from the cinnamon and sugar blend or powdered chocolate that you'll find at some coffee shops. To prevent an insulin response, it's important that you avoid adding any sugar or honey to your coffee. Alternative sweeteners aren't much better since they've been shown to stimulate sugar cravings and potentially increase appetite by activating the food reward center in your brain. If you can't do without a little bit of sweetness, try adding a tiny bit of stevia—it's 300 times sweeter than sugar, so you won't need much! Stevia is a natural sweetener that does not raise blood sugar or promote insulin production. If you do opt to use stevia, it's still important to be on alert for any increase in cravings; just about any kind of extreme sweetness can tempt your taste buds, making it harder to stay on track.

- **Tea.** All unsweetened varieties of hot and cold tea are allowed while you're fasting. Black, green, oolong, and any type of herbal tea are all perfectly fine, but no tea lattes or bottled sweet teas. You can add spices such as cinnamon, turmeric, and cayenne pepper to your tea as well. Same sweetener rules as those listed for coffee apply. A little squeeze of lemon and a dash of cayenne added to your tea is especially good when you have a cold (skip the honey, though).

- **Beet supplement drink.** Beets have a lot of nutritional attributes, but they are also relatively high in carbohydrates so you don't want to eat a lot of them if your goal is weight loss. One way to take advantage of the benefits of beets without having to consume excess carbs is to look for a powdered beet supplement. We created a beet supplement called Primo Beets that we love to drink while fasting because it's low in calories, doesn't have any added sugar, and gives us a lot of energy. It also improves circulation, which is why I love to drink it before a workout (see chapter 10 for more on the benefits of beet powder). Look for any powdered supplement that is no more than 15 calories per serving and contains no added sugar. Whichever one you use, just be sure that you use only water as your "mixer" and not juice, milk, or any other beverage.

- **Greens-based supplement drink.** When you're busy, it's incredibly tough to make sure you're getting enough nutrients throughout the day. That's why we love our Primo Greens, a nutrient-dense, highly concentrated effervescent tablet that you just drop into a glass of water and drink. It's made from blue-green algae, barley grass, broccoli, kale, chlorella, spinach, parsley, Brussels sprouts, and more—and it's OK to drink while you're fasting because it's just five calories and is sweetened naturally with stevia. Any other powdered greens-type drink that is 40 calories or less and contains no added sugar is also OK to drink during your fasting window.

A Day in the Life of an Interval Eater

We've mentioned that when you eat (and when you don't eat) is the most important part of this plan. This simply means that you will want to be sure to eat according to a set schedule. To help you get an idea of how this works in real life, we thought we'd share what a typical day looks like for us. These examples reflect how we might eat when we are following a 16-hour intermittent fasting schedule, like the one you'll follow in this first phase.

Terry

5:15 a.m.	Eyes open
5:30 a.m.	Coffee with nondairy creamer
6:00 a.m.	Start surgery
8:00 a.m.	Primo Beets drink for energy (15 calories)
10:30 a.m.	Hot caffeinated tea and Primo Greens drink for nutrition (10 calories)
1:00 p.m.	First meal of the day: lunch of grilled chicken with lettuce leaves, cut carrots, and pickles (eaten like a lettuce wrap) and a whole grapefruit
2:30 p.m.	Caffeinated drink or beet drink for energy
3:30 p.m.	Snack of egg whites with chopped asparagus
5:00–5:15 p.m.	End of workday; head to the gym
6:30 p.m.	Home
7:00 p.m.	Dinner of grilled salmon with barley and a salad tossed in balsamic vinaigrette
8:30 p.m.	Arctic Zero frozen dessert (an ice cream alternative)
9:00 p.m.	Start 16-hour fast (next meal will be at 1:00 p.m. the following day)

Heather

6:15 a.m.	Eyes open
6:30 a.m.	Beet drink for energy
6:45–7:20 a.m.	Kids up and dressed
7:30–8:40 a.m.	Drop off four kids at two different schools, then head to the gym
9:30 a.m.	Gym
10:45 a.m.	Coffee with nondairy creamer
11:30 a.m.	Primo Greens drink for nutrition (10 calories)
1:00 p.m.	First meal of the day: lunch of seared tuna with miso soup and sliced cucumbers and sprouts with sesame oil and lemon
3:00 p.m.	Beet drink for energy
3:45 p.m.	Snack of cut veggies and turkey slices in carpool line*
7:00 p.m.	Dinner of Petite Filet Mignon with grilled asparagus and zucchini noodles with marinara; "Naked" Baked Apple for dessert (see page 205 for the recipe)
9:00 p.m.	Start 16-hour fast (next meal will be at 1:00 p.m. the following day)

The schedule in the sample days is the one that works best for our lives. If you have an unconventional schedule (i.e., if you work nights or swing shifts), you can move the intervals around to fit your needs. That is one of the best things about intermittent fasting—it's completely customizable to your lifestyle. Obviously, you just have to be sure your refuel interval happens during your "awake" hours so that you have enough time

*Ideally the meat will be sliced from fresh, low-sodium turkey breast at the grocery store deli counter, but in a pinch, I've been known to take the turkey out of a convenience store sandwich and eat that—us moms-on-the-go have to be flexible!

to get plenty of healthy foods into your body. (Because of course you can't eat while you're sleeping.) No matter how you end up structuring your eating schedule, you will want to keep an eye on the end of your refuel interval because this determines when you will eat next. Meaning, if you eat a late-night snack, you will have pushed back your first meal into late afternoon.

Speaking of unconventional, you might have noticed that we don't eat three main meals a day, as a lot of people do (not that we consider a sugary bowl of cereal slurped up in seconds as you're rushing out the door a meal). We aim to eat instead two well-rounded, nutrient-rich meals at lunch and dinner, and then fill in with nutrient-rich snacks as hunger demands. We make sure these meals feature a high-quality protein source that's either steamed or grilled, not fried and definitely not breaded. It's also important to include a variety of vegetables in a variety of preparations, including raw. Vegetables deliver different nutrients based on their preparation, so mixing it up will ensure you get a wider array of antioxidants and other important vitamins. Plus, different textures can add a little excitement to your meals and make your mouth happy. For satiation, we also recommend adding some healthy fats, such as coconut or grapeseed oil, or avocado, and a serving of a complex carb, such as barley or black beans, which I love to add to salads.

In the following food list, you'll discover the specific food options, suggested serving sizes, and number of servings you should aim for during the Red-Carpet Ready phase. If you see anything on the list that you've never tried, don't be afraid to put it on your plate! I remember when I first tried dandelion greens, which I wasn't too sure of, but I ended up loving it.

When you shop for foods, try to get the best quality you can afford or that is available to you. Organic options generally have less pesticide residue, fewer toxins, and higher levels of minerals and nutrients. If you want to be a savvy produce shopper, you can check out the Environmental Working Group's Shopper's Guide to Pesticides in Produce, which separates produce according to levels of pesticide residue. Those on the "Dirty Dozen" list should be purchased organic, while those on the "Clean

Fifteen" list are considered least likely to contain pesticide residue and are OK to buy conventional.

After the food list you will find meal plans for this phase, which we encourage you to use to help you get into a groove with the diet.

Phase 1: Red-Carpet Ready Food List

Proteins (3–4 ounces; 2–3 servings per day)

Eggs
Canadian bacon
Pork bacon (not thick cut)
Turkey bacon
Ham, low sodium
Pork, all types
Venison
Bison
Buffalo
Beef:
- Eye of round roast or steak
- Sirloin tip side steak
- Top round roast and steak
- Bottom round roast and steak
- Skirt steak
- Top sirloin steak

Chicken, light meat only
Turkey, light meat only
Protein powders: whey, pea, or rice
Vegetarian/Vegan:
Tofu (firm and silken; always organic and non-GMO)
Seitan
Tempeh
TVP/soy chunks
Veggie meat crumbles

Fish and shellfish (3–4 ounces; 2 servings per week with the exception of tuna, which should only be eaten once a week due to mercury concerns):

Anchovies
Cod
Halibut
Salmon
Sardines
Sole
Crab
Lobster
Shrimp
Trout
Tuna (fresh or canned—water packed, not oil)

Fats (1–2 servings per day)

Avocado (1/4)
Guacamole (skip ones with added fillers such as mayo)
Avocado oil (1 tablespoon)
Coconut oil (1 tablespoon)
Grapeseed oil (1 tablespoon)
Olive oil (1 tablespoon)

Nuts, Seeds, and Snacks (1/2 ounce; 1 serving per day)

Seeds: chia, pumpkin, sunflower, sesame, poppy seed, flaxseed, hemp seeds*

Nuts: almonds, Brazil, macadamia, pecan, walnuts, pistacios

Nut butter: almond butter (1 tablespoon)

Dairy and Nondairy (1 serving per day)

Feta cheese (1 ounce)

Cashewgurt (1/2 cup)

Coconut milk (1/2 cup)

Coconut yogurt (1/2 cup)

Kefir, plain (1/2 cup)

Parmesan cheese (1 ounce)

Nonfat cottage cheese (1/2 cup)

Nonfat yogurt, plain (1/2 cup)

Skim milk (1 cup)

Nondairy creamer (doesn't count as a serving)

Above-ground** Veggies (1 cup of spinach or other leafy greens, 1/2 cup cooked or raw of all other veggies; 2–3 servings per day)

Alfalfa sprouts

Artichokes

Arugula

Asparagus

Bamboo shoots

Bean sprouts

Bok choy

Broccoli

Brussels sprouts

Cabbage, all varieties

Cauliflower

Celery

Chard

Chili peppers (doesn't count as serving)

Chinese broccoli

Cucumber

Dandelion greens

Eggplant

Endive

Fresh herbs, all varieties (doesn't count as serving)

Grape leaves

Green beans

Green bell pepper

Kale

Leeks

Mushrooms

Mustard greens

Okra

Radicchio

Seaweed

---

*Good source of fiber.

**We'll explain the above-ground/below-ground categories in the next chapter.

Snow peas
Spinach
Summer squash
Swiss chard
Tomatoes
Watercress
Zucchini

Below-ground Favorite Flavor Boosters**

Fennel
Garlic
Ginger
Onions (all varieties)

Fruit (1 cup or 1 small individual fruit; 1 serving per day)

Apples
Blackberries
Grapefruit
Kiwi
Lemon (doesn't count as serving)
Lime (doesn't count as serving)
Papaya
Pear
Raspberries
Tart cherries

Complex Carbs (1/2 cup cooked; 1 serving per day)

Barley
Black beans
lentils
split peas
edamame
Oat bran
Pinto beans
Whole-wheat or multigrain bread (1 slice)

Savory Treats (1 serving per day)

Seaweed salad (1/3 cup)
Popcorn, air-popped (2 cups)
Pickles, no added sugar (1 pickle)
Beef or turkey jerky, no added sugar (1 ounce)

Drinks (unlimited; recommended caffeine cutoff time: 4:00 p.m.)

Water
Coffee
Soda water
Teas
Any "no calorie" drink
No alcohol this phase!

Spices & Spicy Condiments

You can use any spice you would like, but these are some of our favorites:

Basil
Black pepper
Cayenne pepper
Coriander

Spices & Spicy Condiments (*continued*)

Cumin

Himalayan pink salt

Lemon pepper

Turmeric

Spicy condiments: sriracha, Tabasco, harissa, salmbal olek, whole-grain mustard

Spike (Super-tasty blend of spices that I highly recommend! Featured in the recipes for "Southwestern Delight" Salad Pizza, page 167, and Sesame Seed Crusted Seared Tuna, page 185.)

Attention Vegans and Vegetarians

Although we are diehard carnivores, we appreciate and love our meatless friends! That being said, it can be more challenging to find vegan and/or vegetarian foods that offer both higher protein and lower carbs (when compared to the protein/carb ratio found in foods such as steak, poultry, and fish). Soy-based foods will be a top choice since they are protein rich, but be sure to get the organic and non-GMO variety. Tofu, tempeh, and textured vegetable protein (TVP) are all made from soy. Other good options are seitan and veggie meat crumbles, which may be a blend of different types of vegetarian proteins.

For your complex carb choice, you will want to choose beans over grains since they will provide more protein. The beans with the highest protein content are (listed from highest to lowest): soybeans, lentils, split peas, pinto beans, kidney beans, black beans, and lima beans. Be sure, too, to eat a serving of nuts and seeds each day. The best choices for you will be hemp seeds, pumpkin seeds, almonds, and pistachios.

If you find you aren't getting enough food, you might consider adding one additional 1/2 cup serving of cooked beans per day—and this is only if you consistently eat vegan or vegetarian!

Of course, any of these suggestions can be implemented if you are a meat eater and you'd like to try and curb your overall intake of animal products. No matter what your dietary preferences, always keep in mind that the most important aspect of the Dubrow Diet is ***when*** you eat.

Red-Carpet Ready Meal Planner

Phase Length: 2–5 days

Interval Eating Schedule: 16-hour reset, 8-hour refuel

You can use the above food list to create your own meals using this customizable formula:

Meal 1 = 1 serving protein, 2 servings veggies, 1 serving complex carb*

Snack = Whatever you're craving (that's on the list, of course)! A piece of fruit; a quick egg-white scramble; a serving of nuts or jerky; a few slices of deli meat and fresh veggies; a slice of toast with avocado spread on it; yogurt or cottage cheese topped with fruit or nuts—as long as it's healthy, it's fair game.

Meal 2 = 1 serving protein, 2 servings veggies, 1 serving complex carb*

You can also use the following meal planner, which features several of the recipes you'll find starting on page 141. This meal planner will help you get a sense of what you should be eating each day. These aren't intended to be strict and can be shifted around depending on what meals you like most and what leftovers you have on hand. Feel free as well to mix and match; that is, eat one meal from the meal planner and the other based on your own creation from the food list.

Day 1

Meal 1: Grilled chicken breast (3–4 ounces) with 1/4 avocado, a side of pickles, and baby spinach sprinkled with lemon juice

Snack: Fresh berries and walnuts (1/2 ounce)

Meal 2: Baked Salmon Fillet with a side of kimchi (fermented Korean cabbage)

Day 2

Meal 1: Sesame Seed Crusted Seared Tuna with Cucumber and Bean Sprout Salad

---

*You will want to have only one complex carb serving per day; you pick which meal each day is best.

Snack: "Naked" Baked Apple

Meal 2: Petite Filet Mignon or other steak with Pan-Seared Asparagus

Day 3

Meal 1: Smoked Salmon Burrito

Snack: A Savory Smoothie

Meal 2: Easy Shrimp with Cauliflower "Rice," Chinese Style

Day 4

Meal 1: Tri Tip Steak with Basic Chimichurri Sauce and a side of Roasted Tomatoes and Wilted Leafy Greens

Snack: Berries with coconut yogurt (1/3 cup) and crushed pecans (1 tablespoon)

Meal 2: A Tasty Touch of Thai Soup with shrimp

Day 5:

Meal 1: Deviled Tomatoes (2) with a side of sautéed mushrooms and Brussels sprouts

Snack: Grapefruit

Meal 2: Sashimi with seaweed salad

BONUS SUGGESTIONS

Option 1:

Meal 1: Jazzy Gazpacho with 1/4 avocado and 4 ounces of crabmeat

Snack: Apple

Meal 2: String Bean, Tomato, and Turkey Bacon Medley

Option 2:

Meal 1: Bison Meatballs (5) with Classic Marinara Sauce and side of Cauliflower "Rice," Mediterranean Style

Snack: One slice of whole-wheat toast with cucumber, sprouts, and avocado

Meal 2: Baked Salmon Fillet with Roasted Fennel and Wilted Leafy Greens

We encourage you to keep an open mind and be flexible as you prepare meals and snacks. You want to get in a groove with the program. If you try a food or meal that you don't like all that much, drop it from your list and move on to something else—there are too many options to spend time eating flavors or textures that don't work for you. Or maybe consider trying some herbs and spices you haven't tasted before to excite your palate.

No matter how you make it work, keep in mind that *when* you eat is your number one priority. Focus yourself on this first, then on eating healthy foods, and finally on sticking to the right portions and you will be on the fast track to success in no time at all.

Chapter 6

Phase 2: Summer Is Coming

Now that the Red-Carpet Ready phase has given you a little metabolic mojo, it's time to carry forward the momentum into this second phase and ride it all the way until you reach your goal weight. We've called this phase Summer Is Coming—because there really isn't anything more motivating than the looming threat of having to put on a bikini or swim shorts—but you can also think of it as the Get to Your Goal Weight phase.

Since everyone's goal will be different, there is no defined length of this phase. What there is, however, is the option for you to customize the plan based on how quickly you want to see results.

We've created three "speeds" that you can select depending on your personal preferences, and each speed will have specific allowances. We think it's important for you to have options because, let's face it, we're not all the same type of dieter, and too many people fail diets simply because there's no consideration of individual strengths and weaknesses. You can check out the details and make your speed selection on pages 22–23.

In addition to the customized speeds, you'll also find an expanded food list in this phase and the introduction of one of our favorite indulgences: alcohol. If you stretched the Red-Carpet Ready phase to its full five days, I bet you're ready for an adult beverage or two. (I really wouldn't trust a diet that tried to take my brut champagne away from me forever . . .) On pages 87–88, you'll discover the best choices.

Of course, if you are going to get to your goal weight, you have to answer one essential question first: What is your goal weight? If you don't already know, Terry and I will help you figure it out.

Getting to Know Your Goal Weight

I think we all kind of know what our ideal weight is, even if it's not defined by a number. For some people, their ideal weight will be reached once they can fit into that dream dress or slimming pair of pants, or feel rockin' in a bikini. Others will have calculated their goal weight based on a specific measurement, such as the body mass index (BMI). While that is a common weight-measurement tool, we have reservations about it because it leaves a lot out of the equation. Terry has some opinions on BMI and what might be a better way to get the best number for your body.

A lot of doctors use BMI because it's a widely accepted clinical standard, but it's best when applied to a broader population vs. used for an individual to determine his or her optimum weight. It's not the worst way to determine a healthy weight for your body, but it can lead to an unrealistic goal if you have a larger body frame or a lot of muscle (since muscle weighs more than fat). Plenty of extremely fit, muscular people I know would be considered overweight based on their BMI.

The other issue I have with BMI is that body weight is not the only marker of health. There are many other measurements that should be considered as indicators of good health, such as blood pressure, blood sugar or A1C, cholesterol, and even certain micronutrient levels. These tell a larger story, as they reveal how all your systems are working, and not just those that are related to metabolism. Personally, I would love to get a read on the levels of autophagy occurring in my body, but reliable tests for that have yet to be developed.

So, why do we use weight as a marker? Because being overweight or obese increases your chances of developing and even dying from hypertension, type 2 diabetes, coronary heart disease, respiratory complications, stroke, gallbladder disease, osteoarthritis, sleep apnea, dyslipidemia

"You're a Plastic Surgeon . . . Can't I Just Use Liposuction to Reach My Goal Weight?"

Because of my profession, I occasionally get asked about the practice of liposuction and how effective it is for purposes of weight loss, so I thought it would be appropriate to address it here in this book. Even though liposuction is not intended to be considered as a weight-loss procedure, that doesn't mean people don't confuse it for one. Liposuction is designed only for diet-resistant areas of fat, like those stubborn love handles or chunky thighs for which you can thank your grandmother's genes. It actually doesn't affect body weight very much due to a "redistribution" phenomenon demonstrated by fat cells; the remaining cells simply increase their fat storage in response to reduced overall fat cell count.

Since fat is metabolically active, liposuction is likely to trigger some metabolic changes. While there's no scientific consensus yet on whether these changes are entirely good or bad, I suspect they fall somewhere in the middle. Losing fat cells could lower the production of leptin, the appetite hormone that signals fullness and is released by adipocytes (the fancy term for fat cells). If this is the case, you might have less fat on your body but an increased appetite. If you can ride out the discomfort, you'll be in good shape; if not, you might soon be heading back to where you started.

Some research says that liposuction can positively impact factors that affect heart health, such as insulin sensitivity, cholesterol levels, and inflammatory protein levels. But ultimately it's not as effective as diet and exercise at reducing levels of visceral fat, the type of fat that causes the greatest degree of metabolic trouble in the body. At the end of the day, much to the chagrin of plastic surgeons trying to keep up with their overhead, liposuction's sole benefits are really only cosmetic and at most have only weak health benefits.

(abnormally elevated cholesterol levels), and endometrial, breast, prostate, and colon cancers. Weight is also the easiest factor that can be isolated and tracked at home, without the need for doctor's visits or any special sort of tool other than a scale.

As we said, you'll follow the Summer Is Coming phase as long as it takes to reach your goal weight. If your doctor has given you an ideal weight or you already have a number in mind, you can aim for that. We're also providing a chart (based on the Hamwi formula for calculating ideal body weight, created decades ago by Dr. G. J. Hamwi and first appearing in a publication of the American Diabetes Association) that takes into consideration your body frame, which I think is an important factor left out of the BMI calculation.

To use this chart, first measure your wrist. You can do this by wrapping your thumb and forefinger around your wrist, right around where you would wear a watch. If your fingers can overlap, you are small framed; if your fingers touch tip to tip, you are medium framed. If there is a gap between your thumb and index finger, you have a large frame.

Now, based on your height and frame, look at the chart on the next page and pinpoint your ideal weight:

Once you've identified your number, you can adjust up or down by a few pounds depending on what feels best on your body. If you aim for the precise number on the chart and you reach that goal, you can adjust even further; you might discover that you prefer yourself slightly leaner, or with a little more weight.

As you get to know your body better while following this diet, you'll ultimately be able to identify your own metabolic sweet spot, which includes the number you see on the scale and how you feel overall in terms of energy and vitality. For Heather, discovering this sweet spot meant adjusting what she always considered her ideal weight.

More Than Just a Number

I spent a long time chasing a number, only to realize that the number wasn't what made me feel my absolute best. I feel so much better now, even though

Range of Body Weight for Height						
	Female			Male		
Height	Frame size			Frame size		
	Small	Medium	Large	Small	Medium	Large
5' 0"	90	100	110	95	106	117
5' 1"	95	105	116	101	112	123
5' 2"	99	110	121	106	118	130
5' 3"	104	115	127	112	124	136
5' 4"	108	120	132	117	130	143
5' 5"	113	125	138	122	136	150
5' 6"	117	130	143	128	142	156
5' 7"	122	135	149	133	148	163
5' 8"	126	140	154	139	154	169
5' 9"	131	145	160	144	160	176
5' 10"	135	150	165	149	166	183
5' 11"	140	155	171	155	172	189
6' 0"	144	160	176	160	178	196
6' 1"	149	165	182	166	184	202
6' 2"	153	170	187	171	190	209
6' 3"	158	175	193	176	196	216
6' 4"	162	180	198	182	202	222
6' 5"	167	185	204	187	208	229

I'm above what I always thought was my ideal weight. It's crazy how much changes when you get dialed in to the right eating and exercise habits—there's so much more beyond the scale than I ever would have imagined!

Terry is a little different from me in that he is a measurer to the max. He'll never let go of monitoring his weight on a scale, and if he doesn't see the number he's aiming for, it's a failure for him. Although he may not admit it, his *true* measure of success is whether he wants to take his shirt off in public. I know he's feeling really lean and strong when he seems to be looking for reasons to show his hard-earned abs. Even though I give him a hard time about this, he's almost 60 and looks amazing—why wouldn't he want to show off a little?

I mention this in part to tease Terry, but also because it reveals that we all have different definitions of what "our best" looks and feels like. Sure, it's important to establish a number, as this provides a focused destination, but we want to encourage you to also consider what reaching this ideal might *feel* like. Achieving your goal weight is about so much more than just the number; it's a package deal that can come with as many add-ons as you'd like. I'll explain.

Our goals usually have much deeper meaning, if we take the time to look for it. I know when I was working on our dream house, there was the house itself, but there was also what the rooms and the space would represent to our family. I knew the pool would mean years of summer fun for our kids, relaxing times where it was just us, and fun parties with all our friends. I knew the TV den would be Terry's escape ("man caves" are real!), and of course the most important rooms in the house, the kitchen and family room, would be the places we would gather for meals, celebrations, and making memories.

Likewise, when you think about your goal weight, think beyond the physical aspect of this goal. One way to do this is to create a mini "vision board" for yourself, either in your head or on paper. However you do it, be sure to take some time to think about what else your goal weight might represent to you.

Could reaching your goal weight come with the benefit of improved health? Maybe diminish your fears of developing a disease that runs in your family, such as type 2 diabetes? Or, if you have type 2 diabetes or prediabetes, is it possible that reaching a healthy weight could reverse these conditions? (Losing weight has been shown to help reverse the progression of both these insulin-related conditions.) Might weight loss eliminate the joint pain that you've been experiencing since you gained an extra 20 pounds? While I don't know your particular conditions or genetic predispositions, chances are good that an internal and external rejuvenation would improve your health in countless ways.

How to Monitor Your Progress

Even though we encourage you to pay attention to the changes in how you feel while following the Dubrow Diet, those changes aren't that easy to measure, so we do still recommend that you track your weight loss. Hopefully you recorded your starting weight (as we suggested you do before beginning the first phase) and have that stored somewhere in your phone's Notes or in a journal.

Moving forward, we suggest a weekly weigh-in. Checking your weight once a week will allow you to keep tabs on your progress without turning you into an overeager scale stepper. Stepping on the scale too often can be unnecessarily disheartening for women, whose weight will fluctuate more frequently than men thanks to hormonal shifts.

If you opted to track your results visually, you'll want to take a picture of yourself each week wearing the same swimsuit or revealing outfit you wore in your "before" picture. It's difficult to see your transformation when you look at yourself in the mirror every day, but weekly photos can help provide just enough distance so you can really see the full picture.

There are of course other benefits to losing weight beyond health-related ones. There's having the energy to jump up and play with your kids instead of always watching them from the sidelines. There's feeling strong enough to go on a spontaneous hike with friends, or feeling confident enough to get intimate with someone without having to hide your body.

All of this is encompassed in what we would call the ageless effect of the Dubrow Diet. Terry talks about how he feels like he's become an ageless type of person; how at 59 years old he doesn't feel any different than he did at 30 (and I personally believe that he looks better than he's ever looked, but I might be a little biased). This feeling comes from the internal activation of autophagy and the metabolic reset you've likely already triggered by following an interval eating schedule. With consistency, you'll get to experience the ageless effect, too.

As you get started on this second phase of the diet, be sure to think about all the benefits that exist beyond the number you want to see on the scale. Identifying and tapping into other motivators can help keep you on track if you feel yourself sliding off a bit, and it will remind you that the number on the scale doesn't tell the whole story.

Summer Is Coming: Time to Select a Speed

Interval eating, a.k.a. intermittent fasting, has become increasingly popular as a way to eat to promote weight loss. But it's certainly not new. Researchers have been studying it as a "metabolic therapy" for over 100 years, and going even further back, Hippocrates himself noted the use of dietary "purifications" as a cure for certain conditions. And many religions have long been known to practice fasting to help achieve spiritual clarity.

More recently, it's been used by biohackers—people, often techie types, who want to optimize the body's performance using cutting-edge tools and practices—and some doctors who think outside the box when it comes to treating the kind of metabolic dysfunction that leads to weight gain. It's also been used by athletes who want to cut fat from their bodies in the most efficient way.

If you explore it a little bit, you'll discover that there are many ways to approach interval eating. Some people eat extremely low calorie for just two days a week and then eat without restriction the other five. Others fast for up to 20 hours, cutting their refuel window to just four hours. These approaches are a bit extreme for our taste, but they probably work for the right type of person.

Since we want this program to work for the greatest number of people, we've included three diet "speeds" to choose from. The options start with a 12-hour reset window, which is the minimum time you'd need to fast if you want to instruct the body to start burning fat stores, and increase in time from there. Here are your three options, which we introduced to you in chapter 1 but want to reiterate here since you're now in the phase where you'll be using one:

Slow (average weight loss: .5–1.5 pounds per week)

Schedule: 12-Hour Reset/12-Hour Refuel

Comes with: One magical Cheat Moment (snack, side, or sweet) per week

Suitable for you if you: don't have a set deadline for reaching your goal weight; one small indulgence per week is enough to tame your taste buds; 12 is your favorite number and/or you like symmetry; you normally take the scenic route.

Medium (average weight loss: 1–2.5 pounds per week)

Schedule: 14-Hour Reset/10-Hour Refuel

Comes with: One gooey, glorious, get-whatever-you-want Cheat Meal per week

Suitable for you if you: found the first phase of the diet difficult but not too hard; want to see results but don't need to sprint to get them; consider anything less than a full Cheat Meal per week a deal breaker.

Fast (average weight loss: 2–4 pounds per week)

Schedule: 16-Hour Reset/8-Hour Refuel

Comes with: One splendid, splurge-full Cheat Day

Suitable for you if you: want to be just like us (*Us Weekly* style); you want to get to your goal weight as quickly as possible; the thought of an entire Cheat Day makes you want to do a happy dance; you think the shallow end of the pool is wasted space because you're the one who wants to dive right in.

We recommend picking the one that you think will suit you best, but know that you can always adjust as you go, as long as you follow one important rule: don't make any changes midweek. Be sure to complete a full week at whatever speed you've started with, and then shift lanes as needed.

On the days that you cheat, whether it's a moment, meal, or day, you will want to still observe the same interval eating schedule. I doubt you'll have a difficult time determining what to eat when you cheat, but just for fun, I want to share with you how Terry and I indulge.

My Choices:

Cheat Moment: Movie theater popcorn

Cheat Meal: A burger with bacon on a bun and French fries; cookies for dessert

Cheat Day: Breakfast: Eggs with bacon and a biscuit

Lunch: Chinese chicken salad with extra wontons and wonton soup

Dinner: Steak with baked potato, sugar snap peas in butter, pretzel bread and butter; vegan chocolate cake (I don't eat dairy) for dessert with a glass of champagne

Terry's Choices:

Cheat Moment: Potato chips and dip

Cheat Meal: Chips and salsa, burrito with refried beans; frozen yogurt with toppings for dessert

Cheat Day: Breakfast: Frappuccino and a bagel

Lunch: Cheeseburger with bacon

Dinner: Crab cocktail, breaded sautéed fish with tartar sauce, and French fries; cookies and sorbet for dessert

Remember that these are just examples of some of our favorite *indulgence* meals, not recommendations for how you should eat on a regular basis!

Whatever you end up eating during these diet breaks, keep in mind that there's no reason to feel guilty: an occasional increase in calories, especially carbohydrates, is sort of like cross training for the metabolism—stimulating the metabolic functions that regulate sugar and insulin will help keep your system in shape. This should not be confused with encouragement to overindulge—one cheeseburger will hit the spot; there's no need to go for two! If you feel awful the day after, you probably ate too much and will want to modify your allowed indulgence the next time.

Now that you've selected the right speed for your diet, let's move on to the next section—selecting the best types of carbs to get you to your goal weight.

The Four Carbohydrate Commandments

In the Red-Carpet Ready phase, we talked carbohydrates—how they're metabolized in the body and what types you want to avoid if you're interested in preventing the constant creation of fat. It's worth getting to know a little more about carbs, including some easy ways to select the best types for your metabolism and health over the long term.

We call these useful dietary details the Four Carbohydrate Commandments. Read them, remember them, and live them!

1. **Continue to steer clear of factory carbs.** This point is so essential that it's worth repeating *and* is worthy of the number one spot. We talked earlier about the importance of eliminating or limiting your intake of factory carbs, which are the baked goods, cereals, white pastas and breads (made from refined instead of whole grains), etc. that you'll typically find in a box or plastic packaging. These foods provide a surge of glucose, some of which will likely end up getting converted to fat. This is bad, but what's also not so great about factory carbs is that they tend to be low in nutrients, meaning they really don't have much other useful stuff to offer your body.
2. **Select superior fresh carbs: vegetables.** Our favorite fresh carb sources are vegetables. (Yes, vegetables are carbs!) Unlike factory carbs, vegetables provide a wide array of useable minerals and nutrients, including vitamins A, C, D, and E and important B vitamins, such as folate. And they are the best natural source by far of phytonutrients, such as carotenoids and flavonoids. These important nutrients give vegetables their color, and within our bodies they help detoxify and counter the effects of inflammation. We love green vegetables most of all thanks to their high chlorophyll content, which you'll remember can promote weight loss and help lessen cravings for junk foods.

3. **Select superior above-ground veggies.** Even among vegetables, there's a best choice, as far as we're concerned. There are essentially two types of vegetables: those that produce edible parts below ground and those that produce them above ground. You've probably heard these classified another way as starchy and non-starchy vegetables. (I don't know about you, but I don't look at a vegetable and know its starch content off the top of my head—which is why I think it's easier to think of them as above ground and below ground.) Starch is just a type of carbohydrate, so when a vegetable is referred to as starchy, it's because it is higher in carbs and therefore delivers a greater amount of glucose to the body.

   Starch concentrates in the roots of plants, which is why root vegetables—potatoes, beets, carrots, radishes, rutabaga—are the below-ground vegetables you minimize in your diet while resetting your metabolism. Starches are simply large numbers of glucose molecules that have bonded together. So even though you might think you're eating harmless veggies when you consume these foods, what you're really doing is delivering a glucose package that will activate insulin production and potentially derail your dieting efforts. Once you've reset your metabolism, you can incorporate root vegetables more frequently into your diet. For now, gravitate instead toward above-ground vegetables, such as any type of lettuce, spinach, kale, chard, Brussels sprouts, asparagus, broccoli, cucumber, cauliflower, celery, and so on.

4. **When it comes to beans and grains, pick fiber.** Certain complex carbs deserve a place on your plate, and we've highlighted those on the food lists. What makes these choices better than the other options? Fiber. Fiber might be one of the least sexy things to talk about ever, but what it lacks in sex appeal it makes up for in its effect on your body.

   There are two types of fiber: insoluble and soluble. You'll find insoluble fiber in wheat bran, whole grains, and some vegetables. This type of fiber doesn't get absorbed by the body and instead sweeps through the intestines and colon, where it helps remove toxic waste. Soluble fiber is found in beans, nuts, seeds, barley, and oat bran (to name a few sources) and turns into a gel during digestion. This type of fiber has been shown to help lower blood sugar (glucose) and insulin levels. Both can lower inflammation and make you feel fuller after meals, making it easier to stop eating out of habit.

The trick with fiber is that ideally you want to get it from foods that aren't too high in starch, such as pastas and cereals. Your best bet is to get it from vegetables sources, such as artichokes, broccoli, Brussels sprouts, and collard greens, and fruit sources, such as apples, raspberries, and blackberries. And when it comes to complex carbs, top picks include black beans, pinto beans, oat bran, barley, lentils, and whole-grain bread. (It *must* be whole grain!)

The Question of Cocktails

If Terry and I were to have picked up this book, we probably would have turned to this section first. Not because we're outrageous partiers who go out every night, but because we both work extremely hard and, as we've mentioned, we have four kids. (That alone should be enough of a reason!) So, when we get home, get out to have dinner together, or settle down poolside for a bit, we like to have a cocktail, or maybe some wine or sake. This is an adult indulgence that we allow ourselves to enjoy responsibly and in moderation almost every night. (Unless we're in the Red-Carpet Ready phase—no alcohol allowed then.)

Now, you might have heard that alcohol is high in calories and can ruin your dieting efforts. While we can't deny that it contains calories, we can speak from our own personal experience and tell you that it hasn't damaged our dieting efforts. Terry can also tell you a little about some of the research that's come out about alcohol and weight loss and your overall health. Of course, alcohol is not for everyone—if you're not a drinker, skip to the next section on dining out starting on page 90.

We've seen research on alcohol consumption that shows how daily or frequent drinkers have a reduced risk of obesity compared to nondrinkers. This could be due to the effects of alcohol on your metabolism, because alcohol can accelerate metabolic rate and increase body temperature; the production of heat in turn creates a boost in your caloric burn. Moderate alcohol consumption has also been shown to improve insulin sensitivity, which explains its link in some studies to a potentially lowered risk of type 2 diabetes. It's only when you drink alcohol in moderation that your liver readily breaks it down, making it unlikely for negative effects to occur. The same cannot be said for excessive or binge drinking.

The relationship between alcohol and reduced risk of obesity could just be a matter of volume—drinking liquids (with or without alcohol) before or with meals can lower your food intake since you simply will have less room in your stomach. (Or you're enjoying your cocktail so much that the food takes a back seat—I get it!) There's a potential downside to this, of course . . . if drinking more wine leads to you eating less salad, you will have lost out on some nutritional opportunities. If, however, the wine took up space that might have been filled by a triple-fudge brownie, you probably did yourself a favor.

Moderate drinkers were also found in one study to be less susceptible to several cardiovascular diseases when compared to nondrinkers. In moderation, alcohol can lower heart attack and stroke rate by inhibiting the accumulation of cholesterol plaque on the inner walls of the blood vessels. This can reduce the chance an obstruction in these vessels may occur and lead to a sudden disruption of blood flow.

All of this is to say that if you like to drink, you shouldn't feel a need to quit doing so while following the Dubrow Diet. As Heather has stressed throughout this book, one of our primary goals is to make sure this program is sustainable for you, and a lifestyle without the things you enjoy most—in moderation—can be tough to sustain.

The catch of course is that there is such a thing as too much alcohol. Excessive or heavy alcohol intake is damaging to your cells and hard on your liver, and it is also linked to severe nutritional deficiencies, dementia,

Fill Your Glass: Guilt-Free Beverages to Enjoy

I drink water all day long. I fill my S'well bottle and wherever I go, it goes . . . whether I'm in the drop-off line at school, at the gym, or driving up to LA, it's with me. But sometimes I want a little more flavor or a sip of something that feels indulgent without being so. If you have a similar craving, try one of my favorites, such as diet chocolate soda (with a splash of nondairy creamer—yum!) or zero-calorie vitamin water.

Keep in mind that most "diet" or calorie- or sugar-free products are likely to contain artificial sweeteners, such as sucralose or aspartame, or alternative sweeteners such as stevia, agave nectar, xylitol, or monk fruit sweetener. If you need to indulge in something that contains one or the other, definitely opt for the alternative options vs. the artificial—although even with these you will want to keep your intake at a minimum, as they can tantalize your taste buds and trigger sugar cravings if you're not careful.

depression, cardiomyopathy (a potentially fatal weakening of the heart muscle), and several other serious conditions.

If you're interested in continuing with your weight-loss progress and maintaining your long-term health, I'd say no more than one drink per day for women and one to two drinks per day for men is your sweet spot. But don't be afraid to experiment a little, especially if you notice your weight loss has stalled. Try cutting back to one drink or none for a few days, or switch up what you're drinking and see how your body responds. Remember that your overall goal here is to reach your goal weight, so you want to eliminate anything that might interfere with your progress.

We've established that we like to imbibe responsibly, but we also like to do so intelligently. This means staying away from high-calorie, sugar-bomb blended drinks and sneaky cocktails that are flavored with undetectable syrups. And although there are some wonderful beers on the market these days, it's probably best to avoid them as well. (Save it for your cheat day!)

Best choices are brut champagne (Heather's personal favorite); red or white wine; customized cocktails ordered with vodka, soda water, and fresh citrus; or tequila, fresh lime juice, and a little spice. If you're out socially and you've already had the one or two drinks you're allowed in this phase, switch to something like a soda water with fresh-squeezed citrus and a few pieces of mint, or the always reliable and refreshing glass of water. Or you can try one of my favorite combinations, which is soda water with a splash each of lychee, watermelon, and grapefruit juice. You could also buck the trend entirely and socialize sans glass in your hand. This is especially useful if you're about to tell a great story and you want to be able to gesture freely.

How to Dine Out

Making your own meals at home will give you a greater awareness of what you are eating, which is important when you are eating with the intention of promoting weight loss. But you shouldn't have to sequester yourself at home forever, and that's certainly not what we do while following the principles of this plan. While it's best not to eat out during the RCR phase, the rest of the time it's allowed and relatively easy to do as long as you are prepared.

Terry and I like to go out to eat because sometimes it feels like the only chance we have to sit down together and really catch up. I have gained a reputation as someone who tends to order meticulously at most restaurants (surprising, I know). When you're paying for food, I see no problem with getting what you want as opposed to ordering off the menu as is, as long as it's within reason of course. Don't be afraid to ask a lot of questions about preparation and sauces, and be patient with a server if they have to run to the kitchen for answers. Most kitchens have no issues with plating your dish with a heaping side of sautéed green veggies instead of a pile of potatoes.

I manipulate the ingredients to make it lower in calories, high in taste, and as healthful as possible. This used to mean asking for everything to be plain, dry, and steamed, but now I like more oils and more flavor, ideally created with fresh herbs and spices. I've gotten so good at ordering that a lot of the time Terry will just say, "I'll have what she's having."

"Help! I Have to Go to a Brunch/Lunch Event and It's Scheduled Before My Refuel Window. What Do I Do?"

As much as we've suggested that you should try and control your calendar while following our program, sometimes things just come up—you might have to go to a baby shower brunch, an early lunch with your boss, or some other food-focused event that's happening before it's time for your first meal of the day. The truth is, life doesn't stop when you're dieting, and other people don't make plans around your eating schedule or your goals, so you just have to be prepared to make it work.

If you know about the event in advance, the solution is simple: you simply consider your eating schedule the day before the event and make an adjustment. Let's say your event is at 11:00 a.m. If you normally stop eating at 9:00 p.m. so you can have a 1:00 p.m. meal the next day, you would shift the end of your refuel window to 7:00 p.m. and then eat at 11:00 a.m. To get back to your normal schedule, you would resume the 9:00 p.m. cutoff again later that same night. This will technically give you an additional two hours of time during that day to eat, but that doesn't mean you have to automatically eat more than usual. If you notice a little extra hunger, drink a 100-calorie protein shake, or increase your vegetable or salad intake.

Now, if the brunch or lunch is a spontaneous event, here's what you do: you go and you do your best to eat according to our dining out guidelines, and you enjoy yourself without even an ounce of guilt or regret at needing to shrink your fasting window. Sometimes, you just have to go with the flow of your life and then get right back on track.

You can certainly enjoy going out to eat during this phase and beyond, just as we do, but be sure to follow these simple guidelines so you don't sabotage your efforts.

- **Drink a 100-calorie or so shake one hour before you go out to eat.** I like to drink one of our Beaute Shakes, which is made from pea and rice proteins and is sugar- and dairy-free. Both the chocolate and vanilla flavors are 100 calories per serving. If I know that I'll have my first meal of the day at 1:00 p.m., I'll have a shake prepared ahead of time so I can drink it to break my fast. Then I'll go have lunch around 2:00 p.m., often in a restaurant. It doesn't have to be a full hour, but for me this seems just enough time for my appetite to be ready for a nice lunch. Be sure to use a protein powder that doesn't have any added sugar and is no more than 125 calories per serving.
- **Skip the bread and chips.** Having the shake beforehand prevents me from feeling ravenous when I sit down at a restaurant and just diving into a basket of chips or bread. Skip the bread entirely, but if you're at a Mexican restaurant you can do what we do and ask for cut-up cucumber, carrots, and jicama to be served with salsa alongside the chips.
- **Look for protein first, and then add to your plate.** The safest restaurant order is pretty much any protein grilled and served with double vegetables. This could be a steak served with a big side of broccoli, a piece of fish served with sautéed mixed veggies, a chicken breast served with roasted Brussels sprouts . . . and so on. Ask for no sauce or dressings, but use seasonings liberally, along with oil and vinegar and fresh citrus. You could also ask for a salad in place of the extra side of vegetables, but just be sure to avoid creamy dressings.
- **Remember to scan the small plates and appetizers on the menu, too.** Your best option for a meal could be hiding somewhere in the smaller dishes served at a restaurant. You can always order shrimp cocktail as it is, or even ask for the shrimp grilled dry, which is delicious with a little cocktail sauce or just a few squeezes of lemon. Chicken satay is also a fantastic option. Add a cup or bowl of any broth-based soup and a salad, depending on

how hungry you are, and you have a perfect meal. Skip soups that have pasta or rice, and if it's a bean-based soup, just get the cup instead of a bowl. Some of the best soup choices include gazpacho, albondigas (Mexican meatball), miso, tom yum (Thai), chicken tortilla (without the tortilla strips or any sour cream), Italian wedding soup, and minestrone.

- **Peek ahead.** If you're feeling overwhelmed by the prospect of going out to eat and figuring out your order on the spot, take a look at a restaurant's menu online ahead of time. This can be especially helpful if you're starving. Setting your order in your mind beforehand allows you to enjoy your meal without the stress—which is the whole purpose of dining out!

Overall, just make it your goal to order something that will make you feel good *after* you've eaten and not just during the meal. When you follow these guidelines, you should be able to go to almost any restaurant across the country (except for fast-food restaurants) and find a way to stick to the Dubrow Diet.

Ready, Set, Go to Your Goal Weight

The basic eating principles that we shared in the RCR phase are still in place in this second phase. You want to continue to focus on creating meals that include a quality protein, a variety of vegetables, some satisfying fats, and a filling complex carb. Be sure to incorporate some fruit throughout the day, whether you enjoy it in an afternoon smoothie or just on its own. Fruits are rich in antioxidants and nutrients, and many contain fiber, which will help you feel fuller longer. They're also a great way to satisfy a craving for something sweet without delivering an unhealthy dose of processed sugar.

In the next chapter, you'll find the food list and meal planner for this phase. We also encourage you to revisit the RCR Survival Guide on page 58. Even though the tips you'll find there were written to help you get started, they are just as relevant to helping you stay on track through this next phase and the last one.

Chapter 7

Summer Is Coming Food List and Meal Planner

At this point, you should have followed the first phase of the diet for at least two days and no more than five. If you completed the initial part of the plan, it's important to acknowledge yourself for this accomplishment. In just a few days' time, you've set the metabolic stage for increased fat burning and shifted (or at least begun to shift) your cravings away from processed foods and toward healthy and satisfying foods. This is some serious progress—yay, you! Now, it's time to keep a good thing going . . . all the way to your goal weight.

In the Summer Is Coming food list, you'll see additional food and drink choices for this phase. Be sure to take advantage of these by mixing up the meals and snacks you eat each day. This will help prevent dreaded diet boredom, which can undermine your commitment to the plan—let's not let that happen.

If you're a fan of cheese, you'll be happy to see the additions of ricotta and mozzarella, which we use along with other cheeses in our pizza recipes starting on page 163. Since we're staying away from processed carbs, we've put our pie on a cauliflower crust. If you have never tried cauliflower as a pizza base, you'll be pleasantly surprised by how tasty it is. I think you'll like it more if you think of it as a pizza alternative rather than a pizza substitute. (I can't stand when people say stuff like "it tastes just like the real thing" when it doesn't!)

A Day in the Life of an Interval Eater

In chapter 5, Terry and I each shared how our days might look like when we are following a 16/8 schedule (which is the schedule we follow most of the time). Since the diet is so flexible and filled with options, there's no need to copy us . . . especially if you dislike all the foods we love. Just in case you wanted to see another real-life example, we thought we'd share a sample day from Michelle Czycalla from Minneapolis, who participated in our diet test group. Even if her schedule is different from yours, Michelle's sample day will provide another example of how the Dubrow Diet plays out in real life.

Michelle's Sample Day

6:00 a.m. Primo Beats drink mixed with hot water

7:00 a.m. Extra-large cup of black coffee

9:00 a.m. Primo Greens drink (on the drive to work)

12:00 p.m. Spinach salad with grilled chicken, broccoli, cucumber, green pepper, carrots, tomatoes, sunflower seeds with lemon juice and spike spice; 1 slice of toasted whole wheat bread.

9:00 a.m. to 12:00 p.m. 32 oz of water

1:00 p.m. 1 cup of hot mint tea

3:30 p.m. 2 hard boiled eggs and carrot sticks

5:00 p.m. My after work mocktail: 1 glass of sparkling water with 1 tablespoon peach vinegar (similar benefits to drinking apple cider vinegar only peach flavor and surprisingly refreshing).

6:00 p.m. Grilled salmon and steamed broccoli topped with parmesan cheese

7:45 p.m. 1 sliced apple heated on the stovetop dusted with cinnamon

9:30 p.m. 1 cup of calming night tea

Phase 2: Summer Is Coming Food List

The following list of foods can be added to those already included on the RCR food list, meaning all foods on both lists are acceptable during the second phase.

Protein additions (3–4 ounces; 2–3 servings per day)

Flank steak

Beef tenderloin

Chicken, dark meat

Turkey, dark meat

Fish and shellfish

Clams

Mussels

Scallops

Fat additions (2–3 servings per day)

Olives (8–10 olives)

Walnut oil (1 tablespoon)

Almond oil (1 tablespoon)

Nuts, Seeds, and Snacks additions (1/2 ounce; 1 serving per day)

Hummus (3 tablespoons)

Pine nuts

Dairy additions (1 serving per day)

2% Greek yogurt, plain (1/2 cup)

Mozzarella (1/3 cup)

Ricotta (1/4 cup)

2% milk (1 cup)

Above-ground Veggie additions (1/2 cup cooked or raw; 2–3 servings per day)

Acorn squash

Butternut squash

Spaghetti squash

Orange, red, and yellow bell peppers

Below-ground Veggie additions (limit to no more than 1 of your veggie servings per day)

Beets

Carrots

Jicama

Radishes

Rutabaga

Turnips

Water chestnuts (grown under water)

Fruit additions (1 cup or 1 small individual fruit; 1–2 servings per day. Second serving only allowed on days you don't have an alcoholic beverage)

Blueberries
Cherries
Clementine
Mango
Nectarine
Peach
Pineapple
Plum
Strawberries
Watermelon

Complex Carb additions (1/2 cup cooked; 1 serving per day)

Bulgur
Couscous
Garbanzo beans (chickpeas)
Kidney beans
Lima beans
Oats
Quinoa

Savory treats

Nitrate-free salami (1 ounce)
Prosciutto (1 ounce)
Seaweed snacks (1/2 pack)
Smoked salmon (1 ounce)

Alcohol additions (men: 1–2 drinks per night; women: 1 drink per night)

Gin
Tequila
Vodka
Wine

Summer Is Coming Meal Planner

Phase Length: Until you reach your goal weight

Interval Eating Schedule: Customized by you (refer back to pages 22–23 for options)

Week 1 (from Monday to Sunday)

Day 1

Meal 1: Pacific Rim Slaw with a steamed lobster tail

Snack: Nonfat cottage cheese with raspberries and blackberries

Meal 2: Tri Tip Steak with Pad Thai Zoodles

Day 2

Meal 1: Smoked Salmon Burrito

Snack: Ricotta and pine nuts

Meal 2: Roasted Spaghetti Squash with Classic Marinara Sauce and Wilted Greens

Day 3

Meal 1: Shrimp with Quick Romesco Sauce

Snack: Watermelon

Meal 2: Curried Cauliflower "Rice," Indian Style, with lentils

Day 4

Meal 1: Virgin Piña Colada with Benefits Smoothie

Snack: Hummus with carrots and cucumbers

Meal 2: Petite Fillet Mignon or other steak with a simple salad of baby spinach, radishes, tomatoes, and shallots with a dressing of a tablespoon of oil, a teaspoon of red wine vinegar, and Spike

Day 5

Meal 1: Turkey Lettuce Burgers with Onions, Tomatoes, and Summer Squash Medley

Snack: Greek yogurt, almonds, and pear

Meal 2: A salad of lettuce, cucumber, chickpeas, sprouts, avocado, and olives with a simple dressing of olive oil, lemon juice, and Spike

Day 6

Meal 1: Egg Whites, Asparagus, and Mushroom Frittata

Snack: Morning Glory lime papaya smoothie

Meal 2: Baked Salmon Fillet with Roasted Butternut Squash and Wilted Greens

Day 7

Meal 1: Grilled Chicken Breast Tacos with Basic Guacamole and Salsa (Tomato or Tomatillo)

Snack: Peaches and "Cream"

Meal 2: Healthy Hawaiian Pizza

Week 2

Day 1

Meal 1: Tri Tip Steak with Cucumber and Bean Sprout Salad

Snack: Seasonal fruit

Meal 2: Roasted Spaghetti Squash with Classic Marinara Sauce and steamed kale

Day 2

Meal 1: Whole-wheat toast with white fish salad and tomato

Snack: Savory Smoothie

Meal 2: Shrimp with Pacific Rim Slaw

Day 3

Meal 1: Turkey Burger with Red Pepper Tahini and avocado

Snack: Greek yogurt, blueberries, and almonds

Meal 2: Jazzy Gazpacho, salad of seared scallops, strawberries, and arugula

Day 4

Meal 1: Egg whites, smoked salmon, cucumber

Snack: Seasonal fruit

Meal 2: Tabbouleh salad (bulgur, parsley, lemon juice, tomato) with a side of hummus

Day 5

Meal 1: Grilled Chicken Breast with Pan-Seared Asparagus

Snack: Caprese salad (mozzarella, tomato, and basil)

Meal 2: Baked cod with steamed broccoli, dressed with lemon juice and Spike

Day 6

Meal 1: Black Bean Chili

Snack: Hummus with cucumber slices

Meal 2: Siesta Salad Pizza, Apples and Spice and Everything Nice for dessert

Day 7

Meal 1: Egg Whites, Asparagus, and Mushroom Frittata

Snack: Virgin Piña Colada with Benefits Smoothie

Meal 2: California salad (endive, chickpeas, artichoke hearts, peppers, olives, onion)

Week 3

Day 1

Meal 1: Black Bean Chili with ground turkey meat

Snack: Seasonal fruit salad (berries in spring, stone fruit in summer; apples, pears, and oranges in fall/winter)

Meal 2: Steamed halibut or other white-fleshed fish; blanched cabbage

Day 2

Meal 1: Poached egg, smoked salmon, and 1/4 avocado on whole-wheat toast

Snack: Jicama and carrot rounds with salsa

Meal 2: Petite Fillet Mignon with Basic Chimichurri Sauce and Roasted Tomato, Brussels Sprouts, and Sautéed Mushrooms

Day 3

Meal 1: Siesta Pizza Salad

Snack: Hummus with cherry tomatoes, carrots, and cucumbers

Meal 2: Baked Salmon Fillet with Roasted Spaghetti Squash and Wilted Leafy Greens

Day 4

Meal 1: Apples and Spice and Everything Nice (because sometimes you have to start a day with something not just filling but decadent!)

Snack: Steamed edamame beans

Meal 2: Cioppino (a tomato/shellfish stew)

Day 5

Meal 1: Deviled Tomatoes with a side of quinoa and a tablespoon of pesto

Snack: Coconut yogurt with cinnamon and crushed pecans

Meal 2: Cauliflower "Rice," Mediterranean Style, with feta and chickpeas

Day 6

Meal 1: Lettuce Taco Bar—a choice of chicken, steak, guacamole, and salsa

Snack: A Savory Smoothie

Meal 2: Cauliflower "Rice," Chinese Style, topped with scrambled eggs; Berry Tartlets for dessert

Day 7

Meal 1: Avocado half stuffed with crabmeat, drizzled with freshly squeezed lemon juice or yuzu sauce, and spiced with kosher salt, furikake, or sesame seeds

Snack: Seasonal fruit

Meal 2: Sashimi, miso soup, seaweed salad

Chapter 8

Phase 3: Look Hot While Living Like a Human

Congratulations on reaching the third and final phase of the Dubrow Diet! If you are here, you've likely hit your goal weight and you're asking "what's next?" while doing a happy dance, of course. Or, you could be peeking ahead to see what's to come, in which case I'll tell you this much: it's a happy ending.

If you have stuck to an intermittent fasting schedule during the first two phases of the plan, you've probably put yourself right in the metabolic sweet spot that comes with appetite control, increased daily energy, mental clarity, and simply feeling on top of your life game. I see no reason to mess with a good thing, which is why in this phase we want to emphasize generally sticking to the same principles we introduced in the previous phases, with some adjustments that will allow you to enjoy some of the indulgences life has to offer. This phase reflects how we eat now (unless we have an event to prepare for, in which case we jump back to the Red-Carpet Ready way of eating for a few days), and it allows us to maintain our ideal weight, give or take a few pounds.

Reaching and staying at a healthy weight has brought so many benefits to our lives, and we hope you will experience the same rewards. The key is remembering that reaching your goal weight isn't like crossing a finish line; in fact, it's more like embarking on a new beginning, one that will include many healthy returns on the investment you've made in yourself. In this chapter, we will explore some of these returns that will only be more valuable to you as you age. We'll also explain how to adjust your eating schedule for the long term, and what other areas of your life you should take a look at if you're interested in sustained success.

The 12-Hour Fast: Stay Hot and Healthy, My Friends

From now on, we recommend that you follow a 12-hour fast five days a week, while rotating in two days a week of a 16-hour fast. My personal favorite eating schedule looks like this:

Sunday:	12-hour fast
Monday:	16-hour fast
Tuesday:	12-hour fast
Wednesday:	12-hour fast
Thursday:	16-hour fast
Friday:	12-hour fast
Saturday:	12-hour fast

I like doing the longer reset interval on Thursdays because it makes me feel a little leaner *before* the weekend and on Mondays because it helps me recover and rejuvenate *after* the weekend. I suggest starting with this schedule and then shifting the 16-hour days around during the week until you find the perfect eating schedule for your lifestyle.

Maintaining an interval eating schedule is by far the most important aspect of the plan moving forward. This isn't to suggest that you should stop paying attention to what you eat, but we suspect you are already paying more attention to that than ever before. It's not because you are obsessing over calories or stressing out over points or pounds but because you have a new awareness of how your appetite and metabolism work. You probably now notice how certain foods make you feel—i.e., those that make you feel good and those that don't—in ways that you didn't before following the Dubrow Diet, and our hope is that you will continue to gravitate toward those that fall in the first category. (Most of the time . . . Double Stuf Oreos make me feel like crap, but sometimes a girl has got to have them!)

At the start of this plan, we mentioned that part of the goal was to help you develop a sense of dietary direction that points you toward vegetables, proteins, and healthy fats and away from processed carbohydrates. We encourage you to stay on this same path, as not only will it help ensure that you provide your body with the most beneficial sources of fuel, it will also assist in keeping your insulin levels (and in turn, fat storage) in check. Remember to revisit chapter 4 and especially the Four Carbohydrate Commandments on pages 83 and 84 when you need a refresher on the best food choices.

When it comes to how much to eat in this final phase, our hope is that this plan has already given you a renewed connection with your appetite, and that this connection will allow you to eat healthy, satisfying portions without sticking to any strict specifications. However, if you see your weight creeping up or your clothes start to tighten, I would turn your focus first to food volume. Pay attention to how much you're eating, and see if you've maybe strayed from the portion sizes that made you feel your best. If there's noticeable portion expansion happening, try scaling back a bit and see how your body responds.

The ultimate goal for this phase is for you to no longer feel like you are in diet mode, but to feel like you are on the other side of having made a big change in your life. On this side of the change, you are no longer following the Dubrow Diet; instead you are living in a way where your healthy habits have just become second nature. You know when to eat, what to eat, and how much to eat without checking any food list. You've taken the principles of this program and made them your own, and now you are ready to customize how you eat even more.

For a lot of people, the question of customization turns to Cheat Moments, Meals, and Days and how often they are allowed from here on out. Our advice would be to have a Cheat Day once a month and then a

Cheat Meal every other week of the month. But ultimately, it's up to you. If you want to indulge more or less than that, you can do so. Just keep two things in mind: (1) how you're going to feel afterward, and (2) all the work you've put into getting where you are. No matter what, stay connected to your appetite and your body, and don't ignore any messages they send to get back on track.

Creating an Encouraging Environment

There are other areas of your life that can have a significant influence on how likely you are to stick with a behavior change (which is really all a diet is). This includes your friendships, relationships, and career and life goals. When you've made an impressive and profound physical change, taking steps to make the rest of your world as good as you feel can help the change stick.

I'm not saying you have to go out and get yourself a new life or become a totally different person, but I do think it's important that you look at the influencers in your life, and it's especially important to consider how they've reacted to you as you've changed. I am certain that as you've stuck to your commitments and begun to reveal your best self, you've noticed that it has elicited a response in other people. Positive, supportive friends and family have likely rallied around you and encouraged you. The negative complainers have probably tried to drag you down or done their best to derail your progress.

I've always felt that it's easy for people to be friends with someone when the chips are down. It's when you're successful that your true friends will reveal themselves. Those who are happy for you and rooting for you are worthy of the fabulous new you. Hold these people close to you and share your appreciation for their success, too; encourage their efforts to be healthy, kind, and inspirational individuals. We all could do a little more to raise each other up.

Not all your best supporters will be found in your immediate circle. In fact, you might be surprised to discover it's a coworker who regularly comments on how great you look, asks what your secret is or wants to trade healthy recipes, and inspires you to keep going. Or maybe it's that one guy or girl in your workout class who gives you a high five or thumbs-up after your hard workout. Don't overlook these small acts of encouragement! They are momentum bursts, like gusts of wind that can help push you forward if you pay attention to them.

You might consider expanding your circle to make room for people who bring positivity and inspiration to your life. You can also make room by eliminating the constant complainers, but that's easier said than done. In recent years, Terry and I have really tried to develop friendships with people we've met who seem driven and fun, interesting and successful, yet grounded, too. We meet an overwhelming number of people between the two of us, so it's not always easy to see the spark of genuine friendship, but when we notice it, we make a concerted effort to make plans with these people. I encourage you to do the same.

We've also made efforts, individually and as a couple, to jump at opportunities for growth in professional and business realms, even when there's risk involved. For Terry, being on *Botched* meant stepping aside at times from his personal plastic surgery practice, but he considers his experience on the show as one of the greatest gifts he's ever received. He tells me all the time how it gave new meaning to his career and helped him emerge from a bit of professional burnout. Together, we decided to keep expanding Consult Beaute, our skincare and supplement line, even though both markets are remarkably saturated. We do it because it's invigorating to stay connected to advancements in these areas, and because we try so many other products that come out that aren't that good, and we want to work hard to produce stuff that's better.

Endeavors like these are exciting and motivating for us, and having purpose and goals related to them adds a little extra encouragement to stay on top of our health game. We don't have time to feel too tired to fly to Minnesota for a strategy meeting with our supplement team. Terry can't afford to feel sluggish and cloudy-headed because he's been eating junk food for days and skipping the gym, not when he's got a line of international patients on the docket for the week or long days of filming to endure. And I have to be sharp and prepared for interviews, whether it's me who's asking the questions of athletes, musicians, and actors who visit my *Heather Dubrow's World* podcast, or I'm the one who's being interviewed in an E! new segment or other TV show appearance.

So, the question is: Do you have a career or other pursuits that drive you to want to be the best version of yourself, that might motivate you to continue taking good care of yourself? These could be professional or personal. I know that in addition to any professional ambitions that drive me, there's also the lifelong pursuit of wanting to be the absolute best parent I can be. I want to be healthy and happy and capable of doing as much as I can with my kids—and I don't want them to get stuck caring for me if my ailments can be linked to my lousy health habits. (I already feel a little guilty and regretful about the time I spent smoking in my twenties and thirties, but all I can control is how I care for myself from now on.)

You might be wondering: *Heather, what does all this have to do with maintaining weight loss?!* Well, simply put, there's more to life than dieting and losing weight. And we believe that by surrounding yourself with motivators that exist away from the scale, you will also be surrounding yourself with reasons to stay on track with your new eating habits. There's got to be a compelling reason why you want to look and feel your best beyond a darn number staring back at you, know what I mean?

There are also of course hundreds, if not thousands, of health-related reasons that might encourage you to continue to eat well and stay at a healthy weight. Let's take a look at some of the ones that help keep us on track. Although we've covered some of these points, it's worth revisiting them and discovering some additional reasons to stay committed to your new dietary habits.

The Ageless Incentive: Why You Should Stick with the Dubrow Diet for Good

We've discussed the idea of agelessness throughout the book. You've no doubt met "ageless" people before; they're the ones who have that seemingly perpetual healthy glimmer thing going on. You can see it in the brightness of their eyes, their clear, vibrant skin, and in their energy. Ninety-nine percent of the time this appearance is no accident but instead is a product of a consistent commitment to eating well and other healthy habits. (The other 1 percent are those freaks of nature who seem to do everything bad for themselves and still look good.)

The key word here is "consistent"—you don't become ageless by staying on an endless diet-driven roller coaster, where your weight and how you feel is regularly cycling through ups and downs. You become ageless by making choices most of the time that benefit your body and its millions of functions. When those choices include sticking to an interval eating schedule, which regulates your metabolism and helps you stay at a healthy weight, along with the other strategies we've shared throughout the book, you will likely experience a long list of bonus benefits, some of which Terry will highlight for you here.

Better brain function. There's no denying that as we get older our brains seem to change. We lose our keys more often, we forget what we were saying, we can't recall the name of that song from last summer that we played on repeat for months. These could be products of slower-moving neurons or even partly due to the fact that most of us have major information overload these days. Regardless, some research suggests that autophagy can help "clear the brain's cobwebs" by cleaning up broken-down nerve cells. When you intermittent fast routinely and you activate autophagy, you'll also be triggering a form of mind maintenance that could produce noticeable differences in your mental clarity. I know I feel much sharper in surgery and throughout the day when I'm fasting. Fasting can also benefit your brain by helping eliminate insulin resistance, which has been linked to poorer memory function.

Greater stress tolerance and faster recovery. I interact with a lot of people each day, and I hear from so many of them about how stressed they are. If you continue to take care of yourself, meaning if you eat well and you establish a regular exercise practice, you'll be blown away by how much more you can handle across the board. This includes being able to weather challenging times in your life and recover faster from illness, injury, and unforeseen health-related incidents such as surgery.

The reason this is the case is because all stressors on the body initiate a greater demand for resources. Your cells and tissues need more oxygen, more metabolic support from vitamins and minerals, and more "materials" for rebuilding and repairing any damage. During times of stress, sickness, or recovery, your inclination might be to turn to fatty, cheesy, or sweet comfort foods. But sticking instead with your Dubrow Diet go-to foods of lean proteins, nutrient-dense above-ground vegetables, fibrous beans, and healthy grains is a far better bet, as these will help your body recover faster. Is it possible that a serving of your mom's famous lasagna may bring a bit of beneficial soothing, too? Sure, in the short term, but I wouldn't let this lead into a cascade of indulgence.

Better circulation, better sex. When your circulation changes for the worse and you have reduced blood flow throughout the body, this can impact sensation in your extremities and affect genital function in both men and women. In men, a surge of blood is what allows the penis to become erect, and some research suggests that in women, blood flow disturbance may lead to problems with arousal. All this is to say that when your circulation is disrupted, it can lead to a big bummer in the bedroom, to say the least.

Being overweight or obese can disrupt circulation in part by placing excess pressure on blood vessels. There are other underlying factors, such as diabetes, atherosclerosis, and blood clots, that can disrupt circulation and should not go unaddressed. If you've experienced prolonged and/or unexplained sexual dysfunction, you should go see your doctor.

When you maintain your goal weight, you could experience the boudoir bonus of a greater sexual quality of life, not just because you feel better in your body but because your body is simply working better all around. Sex relies upon signals from the brain, healthy hormone levels, and oxygen content in the blood, among other factors. Staying at a healthy weight can help with all of these.

Reduced risk for heart disease and diabetes. As you already know, intermittent fasting and fat loss go hand in hand. This isn't a mystery or a miracle but a product of metabolic science. What metabolic science also shows is that the changes that take place in the body when you routinely fast might reduce your risk for heart disease and type 2 diabetes, two of the most common diseases of our time.

One of the risk factors for both diseases is consistently elevated triglycerides. Your liver makes triglycerides from excess calories and then stores them in your fat cells for later use. Because triglyceride production is tied directly to your dietary intake, you can slow its production when you minimize the intake of inessential calories, something you've already learned to do on the Dubrow Diet by cutting out what we call factory carbs. You can also eliminate calories altogether for an extended period of time, which is what you do when you intermittent fast. This lowers your triglycerides two ways: first, by removing the raw materials the liver needs to make triglycerides, and second, by forcing your body to use fat cells, including the triglycerides they're housing, for fuel.

What the research has shown is that high triglycerides tend to be a marker of some degree of underlying metabolic dysfunction. High triglycerides could indicate insulin resistance, which puts you on the fast track to developing type 2 diabetes, and they are also often accompanied by high LDL (i.e., "bad" cholesterol) and low HDL (good cholesterol), a trio of conditions that is linked to cardiovascular disease. In most cases, triglycerides can be kept in check when you follow a diet that's limited in processed carbs and you regularly practice intermittent fasting. In other words, stick with the principles you've learned in this book!

Sustained ageless internal environment. Earlier in the book, we talked about intermittent fasting and its powerful ability to activate autophagy, your cells' self-cleaning process. You might think of autophagy as the ultimate maintenance phase because when you switch it on, you are essentially deploying a millions-strong team of molecular maintenance workers. This team will work to clear damaged cells and DNA, invading pathogens and bacteria, along with other degraded components of your body. When your internal environment is maintained this way on a regular basis, you increase your chances of staving off disease and premature signs of aging. The catch is that at every millisecond there are metabolic processes happening within the body that will produce waste and damage that need addressing. That means there is *always* more work for autophagy to do, which is why it's essential for an interval eating schedule to remain part of your life long term.

Less panic before big events. This is Heather; I had to chime in here with this point, and I can't trust a guy to talk about it because they just don't relate to event stress the way that most ladies do. I know ultimately this isn't as important as preventing disease, but dress distress can be devastating in its own way. Can you imagine the relief you would feel if you didn't have to crash diet for an event, or if you could open your closet door and know that you could pick out anything and it would fit? Seems like some sort of fairy tale, doesn't it? Well, it doesn't have to be. When you make a commitment to stick with intermittent fasting and a diet mostly free of processed carbs, you'll create a metabolic consistency that will help keep your body in your ideal weight range. This also means staying in the same clothing size range, a relief for your pocketbook and your event-prep process.

Speaking of which, when you get to your goal weight and maintain it for at least a few weeks, it's time to purge! Holding on to larger-sized clothing is like saying in the back of your mind, "I'm going back there someday." If you have things you love, take them to the tailor to make them fit your slimmed-down body.

Of course, this is just a selected list of some of the benefits you'll experience when you stick with the lifestyle changes we've shared with you in this book. These are also some of the benefits that are most meaningful for us, but different rewards might stand out for you, and we'd love to hear about them. If you've experienced a life-changing benefit thanks to your commitment to the Dubrow Diet, share it with us on social media with the hashtag #dubrowdiet.

Taking the Dubrow Diet on Vacation

Since both Terry and I have such long, winding dieting histories, we know a lot about what can make a plan tough to stick with long term. One of the reasons we've both struggled with sustainability in the past is the lack of "portability" with many dietary principles, i.e., it's tough to maintain them when you're not in your usual routine. This is why it was so important that the plan we designed be based on practices that you can implement anytime and anywhere, including when you're on vacation.

Our goal when we go on vacation is to have a great time, but to also not gain what feels like 15 pounds, and to not come back feeling worse than we did when we left. To help with this, we generally try to follow a 12-hour fast on most days we are out of town. In some ways, this is easier when you are on vacation than when you are at home. Here's how we make it happen:

- **Skip the breakfast buffet.** When you visit a buffet, you are more inclined to start your day by overeating and you all but ensure that you won't want to expend any energy after breakfast. I don't know about you, but I want to feel excited and energized to explore wherever I'm visiting. Beginning the day with a buffet is also more likely to help you rationalize eating poorly the rest of the day: "Oh well, I've already blown it so I might as well eat whatever . . ." If it's included in your hotel stay, that's no reason to get off course. See if you can take something to go that you'll have for lunch instead. Most hotel dining room staffs will gladly accommodate this reasonable request.
- **Always plan an activity for first thing in the morning.** Set yourself up for success by having a plan to get moving in the morning. How many times have you puttered for too long in your hotel room and suddenly the day has gotten away from you? To avoid this frustrating feeling, plan a nice walk, hike, or bike ride, or even be ready to get to a museum when it first opens. Start your day with a focus on body movement, not on calories. Even if

it's not in the morning, make sure you get moving every single day. Don't start downing calories until you've paid it forward . . . even if it's just a walk around the hotel grounds or up and down the stairs ten times, if that is the only option you have.

- **If you do end up at the buffet, aim for something high volume and low in calories, and skip the processed carbs.** We always head straight for the omelet station. Order an egg-white omelet with all the veggies you want, and order it dry, which means none of that oily fake butter stuff they often use. This dish will be high in protein and nutrients, but low in the type of carbs that will make you sleepy.
- **Find your perfect vacation drink.** It's fun to get a nice buzz when you're hanging out at the pool or watching the sunset from your hotel room balcony when you're on vacation. But beyond a buzz, you run the risk of ruining a good time for yourself if you pick the wrong libation. We try to opt for a drink that's not loaded with calories but is also tasty and light enough where you can have a few. These days Terry likes vodka soda with a splash of juice or an orange slice, but he used to love those sugary tropical "vacation" drinks! So I made up a trick for him: I look at the drink menu and find the best-sounding fruity, slushy type of drink and ask for just a splash of it to be added to a vodka soda. That was a game changer for Terry; he's completely satisfied without the huge calorie and sugar load. Another option is a tequila and soda with a splash of lime juice, and Tajín seasoning around the rim if they have it. It's spicy and yummy, and you really can't drink it that fast, making it a perfect daytime drink. A spritzer with wine and soda made super cold with a lot of ice is also fantastic for warmer weather. No matter what you choose, be sure that every other beverage is a huge glass of water.
- **Skip the 3,000-calorie salads and overloaded sandwiches.** At just about every resort, you will find overloaded salads and

sandwiches on the lunch menu, often featuring fried foods, processed carbs, and fatty dressings and sauces. If you want to undo some of the progress you've made and/or feel like you need a major diet detox when you get home, go ahead and order one of these options. If, however, you want to feel good on vacation *and* when you get home, opt for something like a burger with bacon and no cheese in a lettuce wrap, or a crudités plate as a snack. Crudités is just a big plate of crispy vegetables, which are perfect for munching on. The goal is to not eat anything that's too filling during the day so that you can enjoy the works over dinner. When we're on vacation, we like to order an appetizer, entrée, and a dessert for dinner, which means our daytime eating has to be especially strategic.

Moving Forward

As you move forward in your life with the habits and strategies you've learned here that will help you maintain a healthy weight, remember that eventually they will become second nature (if they haven't already). Of course, you will have moments where you stray from these habits, but allow for those. There's no reason to beat yourself up; just get back on track, and do it soon before you slide too far back into your old ways. Remember, you can always go back and redo the Red-Carpet Ready phase, which is what Terry and I both do when we need to reorient our eating habits.

Again, the ultimate goal for you in this last phase is to feel as though the diet has really become your own. However, just in case you're still in need of some guidance, we are sharing here a meal planner for a couple weeks. You'll notice that the foods are generally the same, but there are some relaxed parameters: a little more cheese (unless you eat dairy-free, like me), rich proteins such as lamb, a drizzle of honey, an increase in squash, and more below-ground veggies. Remember, these aren't strict meal suggestions; they are just options for you to consider and customize as you'd like.

Look Hot While Living Like a Human Meal Planner

Phase Length: Indefinite

Interval Eating Schedule: 12-hour fast five days a week, 16-hour fast two days a week

Week 1

Day 1

Meal 1: Lamb Lettuce Burgers with tomatoes and onions

Snack: Carrots, cucumbers, and celery dipped in Basic Tahini Sauce

Meal 2: A Tasty Touch of Thai Soup with shrimp

Day 2

Meal 1: Smoked Salmon Burrito with Herbed Egg Scramble

Snack: Greek yogurt with honey and walnuts

Meal 2: Roast chicken (takeout) with a side of Roasted Spaghetti Squash and sautéed leafy greens

Day 3

Meal 1: Lamb Meatballs with "Riced" Cauliflower

Snack: Virgin Piña Colada with Benefits Smoothie

Meal 1: Greek salad

Day 4

Meal 1: String Bean, Tomato, and Turkey Bacon Medley

Snack: "Naked" Baked Apple

Meal 2: Sesame Seed Crusted Seared Tuna with Cucumber and Bean Sprout Salad

Day 5

Meal 1: "Southwestern Delight" Salad Pizza

Snack: Peaches and "Cream"

Meal 2: California salad

Day 6

Meal 1: Taco Bar

Snack: Jazzy Gazpacho

Meal 2: Roasted Spaghetti Squash flavored with olive oil, Spike, parmesan cheese, chopped capers, and parsley; a side of blanched string beans

Day 7

Meal 1: Scrambled eggs with a side of Roasted Tomatoes and Sautéed Mushrooms

Snack: Hummus with rutabaga slices

Meal 2: "Southwestern Delight" Salad Pizza; Morning Glory ice pops for dessert

Week 2

Day 1

Meal 1: Baked Salmon Fillet and a side of Roasted Fennel and Butternut Squash

Snack: Apple slices, 1 ounce of Manchego cheese, and 1/2 ounce of pecans

Meal 2: Petite Filet Mignon and Pan-Seared Asparagus

Day 2

Meal 1: Deviled Tomatoes, steamed edamame

Snack: Banana Grape Chia Pudding

Meal 2: A Tasty Touch of Thai Soup with shrimp

Day 3

Meal 1: Black Bean Chili

Snack: Watermelon

Meal 2: Greek salad with a side of grilled chicken

Day 4

Meal 1: Whole-wheat toast with hummus, tomato, sprouts, and avocado

Snack: Coconut yogurt with blueberries, mango, and almonds

Meal 2: Tri Tip Steak with Basic Chimichurri Sauce and a side of Roasted Tomatoes, Sautéed Mushrooms, and Wilted Leafy Greens

Day 5

Meal 1: Healthy Hawaiian Pizza

Snack: Savory Smoothie

Meal 2: Black Bean Chili with ground bison meat

Day 6

Meal 1: Cioppino

Snack: Honeydew melon with San Daniele prosciutto

Meal 2: Cauliflower "Rice," Mediterranean Style, with chickpeas and feta cheese

Day 7

Meal 1: Sashimi with miso soup and seaweed salad

Snack: Seasonal fruit salad

Meal 2: Shrimp with Pad Thai Zoodles

Part Three

The Must-Have Diet Accessories

Chapter 9

Optimizing the Ageless Effect: The Importance of Exercise

We wrote this book primarily to introduce you to the transformative eating practice of intermittent fasting and so you might also experience, as we have, the benefits that can be brought about when you fast routinely: improved metabolism and the maintenance of a healthy weight, better appetite awareness and control, and regularly activated autophagy, to name a few. But let's say you want more than that. Let's say you want to feel fitter and stronger, even as you age, and you want to improve your energy and mood, in part by countering bouts of anxiety and stress. Or perhaps you just want to increase the fat burning that is already occurring as you follow the dietary principles of the Dubrow Diet.

Well, here's the good news: all of these can be achieved when exercise becomes a consistent part of your life.

Since we're not personal trainers—although Terry did study exercise physiology and keeps himself abreast of all the latest and greatest in exercise science—we aren't going to give you any specific workouts here in this chapter. But we are going to tell you about our own favorite type of exercise and share some of the scientific reasons why you should consider it, too. Plus, we'll offer some strategies for making your workouts happen no matter what. Since this is one of Terry's favorite subjects, he'll get things started.

The Plastic Surgery of Exercise

Early in the book, I mentioned a little about my exercise history and how I used to run dozens of miles a week, training for and competing in marathons and eventually triathlons. I loved pushing myself, loved competing, loved it all. But over the years, I started to find it difficult to set aside all the time needed for this kind of exercise (it turns out that developing a successful medical career is extremely demanding and time consuming). So, I started practicing more efficient forms of exercise, such as lifting weights and running sprints on the beach. These workouts took considerably less time, and I appreciated the improved muscle tone and increased strength I felt.

I liked the sprint sessions so much that I eventually started creating treadmill workouts for me and my friends. These personalized exercise programs consisted of completing short segments of sprinting followed by running at slower speeds, then ramping up the speed, and then back to slow again. They were fast, fun, highly effective workouts. And they represented my first introduction to an exercise technique called high-intensity interval training, which would go on to become by far my most preferred type of exercise.

High-intensity interval training (HIIT) is defined by short, intense bursts of effort interspersed with periods of lower to no effort. As a technique, HIIT can be applied to all sorts of activities, including running, cycling, walking, boxing, jumping rope, swimming, and any kind of bodyweight workout, meaning one that pits you and your body against gravity. A workout of this sort might include exercises such as push-ups, squats, burpees, dips, and so on.

HIIT has become extremely hot over the years, partly because the workouts don't require a lot of time and still produce impressive results, and partly because there's strong science behind it. Here are just some of the benefits that have been linked to HIIT:

- **Increased insulin sensitivity.** This means less insulin is needed for your cells to respond to glucose. This will help you get to fat-burning mode faster during your reset interval and can protect you from developing insulin resistance, a precursor to type 2 diabetes.

- **Accelerated metabolism.** HIIT has been shown to increase excess post-exercise oxygen consumption, known as EPOC. EPOC reflects the increase in metabolic activity (i.e., calorie burning) that occurs as your body tries to return itself to a resting state (a.k.a. homeostasis) after exercise. EPOC levels go up after any type of exercise, but they are elevated even higher and for a longer duration after intense exercise.
- **Increased fat burning.** HIIT has proven to have the potential to burn significantly more fat when compared to steady-state exercise, which is when your effort remains generally the same throughout a workout. High-intensity intervals have also shown to be effective at burning abdominal fat. This fat-burning effect might be due to the fact that HIIT induces a surge of growth hormone, which can help preserve muscle tissue and promote the development of new muscle. Muscle tissue is hungry tissue and the more you have of it, the greater your metabolic burn will be.
- **Optimized ageless effect.** Recent research has revealed that high-intensity interval training has powerful anti-aging capabilities. One study, published by researchers affiliated with the Mayo Clinic in Rochester, Minnesota, found that interval workouts profoundly boosted the ability of mitochondria to generate energy. As we age, our mitochondria—the energy factories found in our cells—naturally lose steam and speed. This can contribute to increased feelings of fatigue and slowed metabolism. What's incredible about this particular study is that it was the mitochondria in the cells of the *older* study participants, who were between the ages of 65 and 80, that produced the greatest improvement, with a 69 percent increase in energy generated. The younger group, aged 18 to 30, showed a 49 percent increase in

mitochondrial ability. Other science has linked interval training with longer telomeres. Telomeres are microscopic protein caps found at the end of our chromosomes, where they protect DNA from damage. Shorter telomeres are considered a sign of cellular aging, which means if you can take steps to preserve telomere length, you should.

These are just a few of the reasons why I think HIIT gives you the most bang for your buck when it comes to exercise and why I've taken to calling it the Plastic Surgery of Exercise. I have never seen another workout technique offer such a healthy package of benefits, which promises to help shape and strengthen your body efficiently and rejuvenate aging cells while also protecting them.

I'm sure you're now thinking, "What's the catch?" And here it is: *high intensity*. You've got to truly bust your butt for short bursts of time to get the most out of HIIT workouts. Though completing any type of interval training will likely allow you to experience some of the benefits I just shared, it will be to a lesser degree than those earned through high-intensity bursts. On the plus side, HIIT is completely customizable in that you are the one who determines what constitutes "high intensity" for you. It's also customizable in the sense that you can pick the activity to which you want to apply the intervals.

Personally, I've seen a consistent commitment to HIIT workouts transform my body along with how I feel each day. I have lost weight faster and gained more energy than with any other type of workout regimen. Plus, my body is much more defined; for the first time in my life (and I'm almost 60), I actually have abs—almost a full six-pack! As added benefits, I've also found that I sleep better and I'm more relaxed during the day.

I've seen HIIT workouts transform Heather's body, too, even though it took some convincing to get her to try this style of working out, which ultimately changed her entire relationship with exercise. I think her experience is something a lot of people can relate to, so she'd like to share more about it here.

Discovering the Athlete Inside

For some people, an interest in exercise comes easily. This is especially true if you grew up playing sports or if your family was active and it was ingrained in you that physical activity was something that should be a regular part of your life. For me, this was not the case. I was raised in a house where you were categorized, and while I became the singer and the actor, my sister, because she played a sport, became the athlete. I wasn't encouraged to find "my sport" just as much as she wasn't encouraged to pursue entertainment. This wasn't necessarily a bad thing, but it did mean that I wouldn't begin to care about exercise until later in life.

It was about four years ago when Terry first told me about high-intensity interval training. He kept telling me about a new gym that was offering HIIT-based workouts, and all I could think about was how scary it sounded to me. I've definitely exercised before and even pushed myself; I've worked out with trainers and gotten really lean and muscular. But I've always had knee problems and haven't ever been into cardio, so I never got into a true groove with exercise. Which is why I was completely surprised by what happened to me after trying interval training.

I'm not going to lie; the first class was brutal. I thought my lungs would explode, and it was *hard*. But when I walked out, I felt like a rock star. Not only did I feel good, but I wanted to go back. My motivation? I wanted to look like the girl who was running next to me. She didn't look skinny; she looked *fit*. When I told Terry this, he said what just about every coach says to a newbie: "Great! Now stick with it." So, I did. I paid for up to six classes a week to force myself into going. I may like to *spend* money, but I do not like to waste it. I knew that putting some dollars on the line was a way to deepen my commitment. (To be clear—you don't have to pay for HIIT classes. You can find a lot of free workouts online that you can do in your own home.) What's crazy is that I started to like it. There was something about the workouts and the structure that motivated me to want to push myself. I think completing short bursts of intensity had a way of showing me what I was capable of—it turns out you *can* push your body to go all out for 30 seconds, and recover enough to do it again.

After three to four weeks of routinely exercising this way, which meant completing at least five approximately one-hour workouts (including warm-up and cool down) a week, I felt amazing. I felt strong, healthy, and fit, and I found the anxiety about my family, career, and other issues that I had been experiencing daily begin to lessen. Research has shown regular exercise to be at least as effective as medication for some people in reducing feelings of anxiety, and that was certainly my experience.

Another part of my experience, and certainly the most unexpected plus to come out of all this, was that for the first time in my life I felt that I connected with the athlete inside of me. I became so charged by the competition with myself, to push myself further, and to feel victory by way of progress that I really felt as if a fire was lit inside of me. (I used to think it was so cheesy when people would say things like that, but I truly felt ignited by my new passion for good, effective exercise. And I still do!)

I believe now that tapping into this feeling is essential to getting and keeping the body that you want, and I believe it is an experience that everyone can have—you've just got to find your "thing." Since Terry and I have experienced such fantastic results from HIIT workouts (and since the research is so strong), we encourage you to give this technique a try. If your ultimate goal is to transform your body, then you really can't find a more powerful combination to achieve it than high-intensity interval training and intermittent fasting.

How to Get Started

The key to incorporating more exercise into your life is that it has to be as convenient as possible for you. The more obstacles that exist, the tougher it will be to make it part of your routine. Here are some tips that helped me create a consistent exercise habit:

- **Try a gym that offers HIIT workouts.** OK, OK . . . you already know this part! But here's how to find a workout spot near you: go online and search for "HIIT gym (or studio, workout, classes, etc.) near ________," and type in your location. Depending on where you live, you may find an entire facility dedicated to HIIT or a larger chain type of gym that offers a few classes. Either way, give it a try.

The Best Time to Work Out

It's often said that the best time to work out is when you'll do it, and this is absolutely true. However, if you want to burn the most amount of fat, we recommend that you work out in the mornings or at some point before you eat your first full meal. If you're following an interval eating schedule, by the time morning rolls around, you will have already fasted for a significant number of hours and your body will likely be burning through the last of its glycogen stores and moving on to burning fat as fuel. If you complete a workout during this metabolic window, you will increase the transition to fat and the burning of fat stores. Did you get that? If you work out during this window, you will basically *burn more fat*!

If you exercise before a meal, you will also have higher levels of adrenaline in your system, which means more energy for your workout, and increased growth hormone, which will help you preserve and build fat-burning muscle tissue.

I know: it sounds counterintuitive to exercise—especially at "high intensity"—on an empty stomach. But the fact is, you won't know how you will respond to exercise in a fasted state until you've tried it. For this reason, you may want to start with a less-intense workout to see how you feel during and after each session. While your body will get better at burning fat as fuel over time, when you first practice intermittent fasting, you may feel a little sluggish during your workouts, even with the increase in adrenaline. If over time you still don't feel supercharged and strong when you exercise in a fasted state, consider increasing your water intake to ensure you're properly hydrated. You can also try adding a caffeine gel shot before working out. I like the little 50-calorie GU packets; they're a great source of non-jittery caffeine that don't bother my stomach and give me a little boost of energy. Since they're low calorie, they won't disrupt your fasting cycle (this isn't to say they are healthy, but they do help with energy).

- **Find a place that's close to your home or work.** If you find a couple options, pick the most convenient location. I ended up going to a place that's right across from Terry's surgery center and near the kids' school, so that was a win-win. I've had friends try to talk me into going to their favorite gym across town or just the next town over, but I *know* convenience is an absolute priority for me. My schedule is just too packed to have to add extra time to get to where I need to be. If you're the same way, pick a spot that's close to you! If you can't find a group class near you, you can find plenty of at-home workouts online to get you started, most of which require no equipment. Simply type "HIIT workouts" into Google and perform a search. Then pick one you'd like to try.

- **Get a comfortable workout outfit (and buy multiples of what works).** It's important to feel comfortable when you work out, so put in the time to find something that fits you and "moves" well, meaning it doesn't feel too tight or restricting. (I also think you should love how you look, but that's just me.) When I found the outfit combo I liked, I bought multiples because I'm sort of a creature of habit. I wear Lululemon pants, a Lorna Jane workout bra, and a Forever 21 tank top with HOKA One One shoes. I wear it so often that my seven-year-old Coco once said to me, "You wear the same outfit every day!" I work out after I drop them at school, so she thinks I don't change, but this outfit has simply become my workout "uniform."
- **Have your workout clothes prepared the night before.** This sounds like such a no-brainer, but it's proven to be extremely helpful with sticking to my workouts. When I get home from the gym, the first thing I do is dump out the old stuff from my bag and throw in the new stuff. I put in my fresh workout outfit, clean socks, and a towel. You restock your workout bag just like you might pack your kids' lunch for the next day. Mornings at our house are usually chaotic and unpredictable, which is why I've learned that if I leave my workout prep stuff until the morning, it does not work. Put your bag with all your clean stuff and your sneakers by the door and make sure you're ready to go.

- **Create a playlist of songs that motivate you.** The gym I've been going to plays their own music, but when I head out to do anything on my own, I always have some good music to listen to. The best workout songs for me are the ones I can sing and dance to, the songs that make me want to move. My favorite playlist would include music from artists like Britney Spears, Lady Gaga, Pink, Gucci Mane, Madonna, Queen, Foreigner, Selena Gomez, and Katy Perry. You can also download a favorite podcast or audiobook, which can provide a good distraction that might help take your mind off how hard you're working. If you're looking for a new favorite podcast, be sure to check out *Dr. and Mrs. Guinea Pig* with Terry and me, and my podcast *Heather Dubrow's World*. Both are available on iTunes.
- **Have a goal to get daily exercise.** I know this might sound like a lot, but this doesn't necessarily mean that you have to get in a full-blown workout every day. It's more about establishing a mindset in which getting some type of physical activity every day is important. You can take your kids or your dog on a hike or longer walk. You can go swim in the pool for a bit, if you have access to one. Walk up and down the stairs in your house, or do some lunges through the living room. If you've been sitting for a long time, stand up and do some jumping jacks or run in place, or turn on some music and dance around a bit. The key is that you want to start to do things that are more active rather than sedentary; there's always something you can do. If you're saying "I don't have the time," that's simply not true. Anyone can grab a jump rope for five minutes (try 30 seconds of jumping, followed by 30 seconds of rest; repeat five times) or do a quick at-home circuit of 10 squats, 10 push-ups (on your knees if needed), and 10 sit-ups. You can complete three rounds of these in less than seven minutes.

- **No matter what, show up, and give yourself kudos for doing so.** When I can, I like to take my 14-year-old daughter Max with me to the gym. Sometimes she does great, and other days she doesn't really put a whole lot of effort into it, and she seems to feel a little disappointed in herself. I think we all feel this way at times, but what I tell her and what I tell myself and what I'm telling you is that the most important thing of all is showing up in the first place. Working out is now part of the fibers of my being, and what I'm most proud of is that I don't settle anymore for excuses like "I'm too tired" or "maybe I'll go this afternoon" or "I'm too busy to go work out." I have made the commitment to take care of myself, and I'm not ever going to back away from this promise. So what if some days you feel like a million bucks and other days you feel like crap! You showed up, you did what you could do, and sometimes that's just enough. Walking in the door is half the battle.

In Praise of Movement

All this talk of exercise and high-intensity training can be boiled down to a simple concept: movement. No matter what your starting point, the most important movement goal you should have for yourself is to just start doing more of it. I have found that as a general rule, the more you move, the more you'll want to move, and the more you feel uncomfortable *not* moving. When you work out your muscles and break a sweat on a consistent basis, your body begins to crave physical activity and the cleansing, invigorating power of exertion—so much so that you will find it practically pushing you out the door.

I guess what I'm saying is, what are you still doing here reading this page? Go get your workout in! (And then do it again tomorrow.)

Chapter 10

Give Yourself a Boost: Supplemental Support

It's time to talk a little bit about supplements. We have plenty of people call into our *Dr. and Mrs. Guinea Pig* podcast asking about supplements, so we know there are a lot of questions out there on this topic. People often ask if we take supplements personally, or if they should take them, and if so, which ones? They often specifically want to know if it's good to take a multivitamin every day. The short answers to these questions are:

1. Yes.
2. We think so, but ultimately it's up to you and your doctor.
3. We have some favorites.
4. Yes, this includes a multivitamin.

If you want the longer answers, keep reading!

In this chapter, we'll share with you some of the supplements we love and what type of support they may be able to offer your body while you're following the Dubrow Diet and beyond.

The Role of Supplements

In an ideal world, your diet would provide all the vitamins and minerals you need to function at your best. Real food is the best source of most nutrients, and it's the one that your body prefers. Unfortunately, what the research shows is that the typical American diet is lacking in a lot of essential nutrients. As you eliminate processed foods and incorporate more quality lean proteins, nutrient-rich greens, and fibrous grains, you'll replenish some of these nutrients that may have been dipping a bit low. Still, even with those changes in place, it's tough to get enough of everything you need across the board. That's where supplements come in.

I only recently came around to the idea of using supplements. In fact, I used to roll my eyes when my friends would pull out a little pillbox or baggie of vitamins that they needed to take throughout the day. I generally believed that it was possible to eat well enough to keep all your systems running, and that supplements weren't worth the time or money.

That all began to change when I experienced severe hair loss after my last pregnancy. I had always had thick, amazing hair, and it was suddenly so thin that I could barely stand it. I ended up taking biotin, a type of B vitamin, to help with hair regrowth and it was like a miracle; after three months or so, my hair was back to normal. This marked the first time that I started to think maybe there was something to this supplement stuff.

The other thing that happened to make me reconsider supplements was that I started aging. (Shhh, don't tell anyone!) And I felt like I was in a position where I was ready to ramp up what I was offering my body. I continued taking biotin even after my hair health had been restored, then added a multivitamin, and then CoQ10 and some others. These days I have my own pill container . . . and I should probably say sorry to those people I had judged just a tiny bit before.

I can say that I feel healthier than I've ever felt, and the collection of habits in my life at this point includes taking supplements every single day. I'm not about to mess with the good thing I have going, so I guess I will just have to continue to make room in my purse for that little container. (I like the ones that are marked for each day of the week separated into a.m. and p.m.)

Since Terry is the doctor in the family, he is going to give you details on some of the supplements we like. That being said, these are not prescriptions, and you should always be sure to consult with your own physician before taking any new supplement.

Our Six Favorite Supplements

As Heather pointed out, most people have dietary gaps that will leave them potentially low or deficient in certain nutrients. I believe this to be true no matter how well balanced your diet and exercise program; you simply can't get the proper daily requirements of important nutrients and vitamins to support all the physiological systems of the body. This is even more so the case when you're following any type of plan that encourages weight loss, such as the Dubrow Diet, because the metabolic demands become greater. As your metabolism increases, your body can become depleted of the energy-producing enzymes and cofactors required to sustain yourself during periods of weight loss. (A cofactor is anything that works with something else to bring about an effect.) Supplements can help meet the increased demands and prevent depletions.

Since supplements are not regulated by the US Food and Drug Administration (FDA), it is important to get them through a reputable source, preferably manufactured at well-regarded laboratories known for quality control. Otherwise, you might not be getting what you think you're paying for. A study published in 2013 found that out of 44 herbal products tested, most contained a lot of "product substitutions" and/or fillers. Generally speaking, it's a good idea to buy products made in this country and avoid those making claims that are too good to be true. With those guidelines in mind, let's take a look at our supplement favorites.

1. **Multivitamin.** Multivitamins are important during weight-loss regimens and beyond in order to maximize the function of all your organs and energy systems. A well-balanced multivitamin should contain not only a full complement of essential vitamins

but collagen, hyaluronic acid, and antioxidants in order to maximize your health, wellness, and beauty (and that includes the health, wellness, and beauty of your hair, skin, and nails).

2. **Vitamin D3.** Research that has come out over the past decade has expanded our understanding of the importance of vitamin D. This fat-soluble vitamin has long been known for its role in helping the body absorb calcium, making it essential for strong bone growth, and a deficiency in D has been linked to increased risk for developing osteoporosis. What's more surprising of late is the research that's come out connecting vitamin D deficiency to increased risk for everything from cardiovascular disease to autoimmune disease to certain types of cancer. This suggests that it is important to many functions and systems throughout the body, and ensuring that you have healthy levels of it should be a priority.

   Vitamin D can be obtained from food, with the best dietary sources being wild-caught salmon, herring, and canned tuna. If you do want to boost your dietary intake of D, get it from these foods and not from the packaged and processed ones that are marked with a "Vitamin D Enriched" label. (Remember, processed foods are a no-no on the Dubrow Diet.)

   Vitamin D can also be created by the body, specifically in the skin when it's exposed to sun. Sun exposure activates the synthesis of vitamin D, and from there it will go on to be metabolized in the liver and kidneys. In theory, if you get enough sun, you should not be low in vitamin D. However, most people today either don't spend enough time in the sun to allow for sufficient production to take place, or they wear sunscreen, which blocks the ultraviolet rays needed for D synthesis. You would need 15 minutes of sun a day *without sunscreen* and with a decent amount of exposed skin to generate adequate levels of vitamin D in the body. While wearing sunscreen and limiting sun exposure are necessary to protect against skin cancer, they do seem to have had the unintended consequence of limiting our bodies' natural ability to regularly replenish stores of vitamin D. This is where supplementation comes in.

If you want to start taking a vitamin D supplement, opt for the "D3" variety, as this has proven to be the most potent form. You could get your levels checked by your doctor beforehand so that you have a marker by which to gauge the impact of the supplement. Just know that it takes a little while to bump your levels up—at least 30 to 40 days. I like a dosage of about 3,000 to 5,000 IU, but your doctor might recommend a different dosage depending upon your current levels.

3. **Coenzyme Q10 (CoQ10).** CoQ10 is an essential antioxidant made in the liver that's used by every cell in the body. Your cells contain organelles—specialized parts of the cell that essentially function like organs—and the main organelle is our old friend mitochondria. Within mitochondria a reaction occurs that produces adenosine triphosphate, or ATP, the life force that powers all functions within the body. CoQ10 is the cofactor that allows this vital reaction to take place. It's pretty important stuff, to put it mildly.

   You can get CoQ10 in some foods, such as beef and chicken, but it's difficult to get enough from diet alone. Levels of CoQ10 decline as we age, so much so that typically at age 40, you'll have half the amount you had at 20. As the level goes down, your ability to make ATP diminishes. CoQ10 levels can also be lowered by certain medications, including statins, which severely lower this vital antioxidant. For this reason, I think that everybody who is on a cholesterol-lowering medication should be taking 200 milligrams (mg) of CoQ10 a day.

   Beyond that, I really believe that just about anyone over the age of 35 should be taking this supplement. The most concentrated levels of CoQ10 are found in the heart, and just like in the rest of the body, your heart cells lose the ability to use it to make

ATP as they age. Declining levels of ATP can lead to less-efficient heart function, weakened heart muscles, high blood pressure, and ultimately, if not controlled or corrected, congestive heart failure.

The strongest research to come out on CoQ10 is related to heart health. Studies have found that taking CoQ10 is associated with improved heart function, and in people with heart failure, it is proven to help them start feeling better. It has also shown promise in the areas of kidney disease and Alzheimer's disease. I personally appreciate the fact that CoQ10 can help neutralize the production of free radicals that occurs as energy is produced. Since free radicals can cause cellular damage and advance the aging process, taking steps to combat them is always warranted.

You can maximize the absorption of CoQ10 by looking for one that contains piperine, an extract derived from the pepper plant. Piperine makes CoQ10 more bioavailable, meaning it increases its absorption, and it can amplify and augment the CoQ10's effect on the cells. Look for a brand of CoQ10 that provides a 200 mg dose and contains 5 mg of piperine (you might see this appear on a supplement label as "BioPerine").

4. **Biotin.** Biotin is a water-soluble B vitamin that you might also see by the name B7. It plays an important role in metabolism, as all B vitamins do, by helping your cells convert carbohydrates, fats, and proteins into usable fuel. You can get biotin from foods, with beef liver providing the highest amount. Other dietary sources include whole eggs, salmon, and sweet potatoes.

   A deficiency in biotin can lead to problems such as hair loss or brittle nails and may even cause skin rashes to develop. As Heather mentioned, she credits biotin with helping restore her hair health after pregnancy, and her positive experience is reflected in research, which has shown that supplemental biotin can help improve hair growth and increase hair strength. While true deficiencies are rare, biotin can improve the structural integrity of keratin, the main protein that forms your hair, nails, and skin. Making sure you have enough of it then could improve the appearance of all these beauty markers.

I like taking biotin for its support of enzymes important to metabolism. There is also some research that shows that when combined with chromium picolinate, biotin can improve blood sugar levels in people with type 2 diabetes. This further validates its influence on metabolic functions, which we know we want to support as much as possible during weight loss.

Look for a biotin supplement that offers 8,000 micrograms.

5. **Beet Supplement.** Beets are root vegetables that are high in folate, manganese, and potassium and are also a good source of vitamin C. They also contain betalains, which are phytonutrients known to have antioxidant and anti-inflammatory properties. Impressive stats, but we haven't even gotten to my favorite beet characteristic, and that's its high bioavailability of dietary nitrate. Dietary nitrates are bonds of nitrogen and oxygen found in certain foods that are converted in the body to nitrites, which are then converted to nitric oxide (NO).

   You may have heard of NO as something that's used in workout supplements. People started using it this way because it stimulates a process called vasodilation. During vasodilation, the blood vessels relax and open up, which increases the delivery of oxygen-rich blood cells. The blood cells can then travel faster and more efficiently to the parts of the body where you need them most. When you're working out, the extra influx of oxygen can increase your overall energy level and performance potential—muscles love fresh oxygen.

   You don't have to be working out to experience the energizing effect of NO. The cells that line your blood vessels, called endothelial cells, produce nitric oxide naturally, and this helps keep your bloodstream moving. When you add supplemental NO, you can potentially increase the amount of oxygen and energy available to the body. Because nitric oxide is a short-lived gas, the effect is only temporary.

In recent years, beets in supplement form (i.e., highly concentrated) have shown promise as one of the best ways to deliver NO to the body, perhaps thanks to its many other nutritional benefits. Preserved meats also contain nitrates, but these are delivered alongside an unhealthy dose of sodium. Beet-derived supplements have been shown to help reduce blood pressure, reduce inflammation, and protect endothelial function. Look for a supplement that uses both the beet leaves and root, and ideally includes some additional anti-inflammatory ingredients.

6. **Greens-based Supplement Drink.** Some of the most powerful phytonutrients and antioxidants are found in green leafy plants, such as spinach, kale, and parsley, and in other green veggies, such as broccoli and Brussels sprouts. The problem is that most of us don't take advantage of all the benefits these foods have to offer because we don't include enough of them in our diets. In fact, according to the US Department of Agriculture (USDA), the average American eats less than half of the recommended amount of vegetables every day, and only 10 percent of what we do get down is the most nutritious green type. (Side note: Do you know what the most commonly consumed vegetables are in the United States? Potatoes and tomatoes, mostly in the form of French fries and ketchup.)

   The best way to increase your intake of the nutrients found in green veggies is of course to consume more of the vegetables themselves. We hope that as you follow our plan, this will happen naturally as you look to fill your plate with nutrient-dense fresh foods. Another way to increase your intake is to take a quality greens-based supplement. A greens-based supplement is able to provide a significant amount of nutrients in a highly concentrated form. Some of these might come as a powder or an effervescent tablet, both of which you would add water to and then drink. Ideally, find one that can offer you some of the nutrients from the types of greens you might not normally eat (simply scan the supplement's ingredient list to see if it includes greens that are missing from your diet).

We recently came out with a greens supplement from Consult Beaute called Primo Greens. We like it because it's only five calories, contains no added sugar, and includes the superfoods spirulina, matcha tea, aloe leaf extract, blue green algae, and chlorella, in addition to several other green vegetables. If you try it, let us know how you like it! Of course, there are plenty of other options on the market, but just be sure you get one that doesn't have any added sugar and is low in calories—especially if you are going to drink it during your fasting window.

It's important to keep in mind that supplements aren't magic bullets, and that in most cases, it could take between 30 and 90 days for you to experience any noticeable effects. How quickly you notice any benefit could also depend upon your levels of each vitamin and mineral before you start. That is, if you are deficient or borderline deficient in any specific supplement, it may take longer to see or feel results. Be sure to continue to prioritize eating a variety of fresh, nutrient-rich foods, as this will also be key to replenishing low vitamin and mineral levels.

Chapter 11

Cheers to You (and Your Bright Future!)

It's hard to know what to say at the end of a book like this when you feel as if you've gone through a journey together. More than anything, we want to thank you for trusting us to give you guidance and to share our insight with you across these pages. It has been our pleasure, and we truly hope that what we've shared here has brought positive changes to your life.

Of course, this doesn't mean that your journey in the pursuit of a healthy life is over, and inevitably there will be times that challenge your commitment to the habits that you know make you look and feel your best. What's important is that you make a promise to yourself that slipups won't become full-blown backslides into unhealthy habits. If you veer off course, simply acknowledge it, and then take steps to self-correct. One reliable way to accomplish this is to do a repeat of the Red-Carpet Ready phase. You might also consider that maybe your slipup was partly the result of boredom? If so, we suggest taking a look at what you're eating and how you're exercising and consider mixing things up in one or both departments. Try some recipes or foods you haven't tried, or maybe even take a healthy cooking class. As for exercise, check out a new workout class or recruit a workout buddy for additional encouragement and accountability. And always be on the lookout for other ways you can add a little excitement to your health journey!

While this marks the end of *The Dubrow Diet*, this doesn't have to be the end of our time together. We hope you'll stay in touch with us on social media. Here's where you can find us:

Heather:

On Instagram, Twitter, and Facebook: @heatherdubrow

Website: heatherdubrow.com

Terry:

On Instagram, Twitter, and Facebook: @drdubrow

Website: drdubrow.com

We would love to see your before and after pictures and hear your success stories, or you can submit questions to be answered by us on our *Dr. and Mrs. Guinea Pig* podcast. We look forward to hearing from you! Until then, keep making your health a priority, be sure to continue to cultivate a solid support group, and remember to have fun! These are three investments that will forever give back to you.

The Dubrow Diet Recipes

We hope you enjoy the recipes we're sharing in this section, which have been created using some of our favorite ingredients. These recipes were designed specifically to help you prepare at-home meals that are directly in line with your weight-loss and weight-maintenance goals. They do not require advanced cooking skills, a daring palate, or excessive investment of time.

To help make cooking easier, pick a weekly grocery shopping and meal prep day. Write a shopping list based on the ingredients of any recipes you want to try, and include other items from the food lists that you might need over the next four to five days. Go shopping, get yourself home, and then get to prepping (preferably with some good music on). This could mean washing and chopping lettuce for salads; dicing a couple onions; slicing or shredding cabbage; cutting up cauliflower, broccoli, and zucchini; and storing everything in the fridge for later use. You could also prep a few small "to go" bags with fresh-cut veggies and some sliced turkey. This shopping and prep day doesn't have to be the day you do a lot of cooking, too, but getting some of the preparation out of the way will help cut down on cooking time and any related stress. Plus, it's kind of fun to have containers of pre-prepped stuff—it makes you feel like a professional chef!

Since we like family-friendly meals in our household, you'll see a couple "make your own" options such as the burger and taco bars, a healthy pizza night with a twist, and an egg-centric breakfast. Some recipes are capable of doing double duty. Raw burger mixes, for instance, can easily be converted to meatballs, and some of our smoothies are naturally sweet and dense enough to be enjoyed as a dessert. Some dishes—like the chili and condiments—can be made in bulk and frozen. The ingredients we use can be found on the shelves of your local supermarket, and the dishes we are offering are easy to mix and match for the pickier eaters in your family. These meals are meant to be enjoyed without the overload of carbohydrates that are so prevalent in the standard American diet. Our main goal here is to help you attain balanced blood sugar (so you can get into fat-burning mode faster during your reset intervals), which will help you lose and later maintain ideal weight.

You'll see that some recipes include a phase note after the title (e.g., Phase 2 only), which means you'll only want to enjoy it after you've reached the specific phase noted. Also, you may see some ingredients included here that aren't on the food lists. This is because once the ingredient is spread out over an entire recipe, the amount per serving is very small.

We hope you find some recipes to love here—please let us know at #dubrowdiet if you discover any new favorites!

Anytime Egg Dishes

Egg Whites, Asparagus, and Mushroom Frittata
Smoked Salmon Burritos with Herbed Egg Scramble and Avocado Stuffing
Deviled Tomatoes

Burger Bar, Three Ways

Burgers

Bison Burger Patties
Turkey Burger Patties
Lamb Burgers

Burger Toppings

Bell Pepper and Onion Topping for Bison/Beef Burgers
Onion, Tomato, and Summer Squash Medley for Bison/Beef burgers
Basic Tahini Sauce
Red Pepper Tahini Spread for Turkey Burgers

Taco Bar, Three Ways

Taco Fillings

Tri Tip Steak

Grilled Chicken Breasts

Easy Shrimp for Tacos, Shrimp Cocktail, or Salad Toppings

Taco Toppings

Tomatillo Salsa

Roasted Tomato Salsa

Basic Guacamole

Pizza Night, Three Ways (Phase 2 only)

Cauliflower Pizza Crust

The Siesta Salad Pizza

The "Southwestern Delight" Salad Pizza

Healthy Hawaiian Pizza

Superstar Veggie Dishes

String Bean, Tomato, and Turkey Bacon Medley (side or main dish)

Roasted Tomato, Wilted Leafy Greens, and Sautéed Mushroom Platter

Roasted Brussels Sprouts

Roasted Fennel, Brussels Sprouts, and Butternut Squash

Pan-Seared Asparagus

Cucumber and Bean Sprout Salad

Pacific Rim Slaw

"Riced" Cauliflower

Cauliflower "Rice," Chinese Style

Curried Cauliflower "Rice," Indian Style

Cauliflower "Rice," Mediterranean Style

Main Meal Proteins

Petite Filet Mignon

Baked Salmon Fillets

Sesame Seed Crusted Seared Tuna

Classic Meatballs

Squashes, Soups, and a Chili, Too

Pad Thai Zoodles

Roasted Spaghetti Squash

A Tasty Touch of Thai Soup

Jazzy Gazpacho

Black Bean Chili

Sauces

Basic Chimichurri Sauce

Classic Marinara Sauce

Quick Romesco Sauce

Smoothies and Desserts

A Virgin Piña Colada with Benefits Smoothie

A Savory Smoothie

Morning Glory (lime papaya smoothie or ice pops)

Banana Grape Chia Pudding (smoothie or dessert)

Peaches and "Cream"

A Berry Tartlet

"Naked" Baked Apples

Apples and Spice and Everything Nice

Anytime Egg Dishes

Egg Whites, Asparagus, and Mushroom Frittata

Enjoy this protein-packed frittata (a fancy name for an unfolded omelet) anytime of day. We recommend using an electric mixer to whisk the egg whites to make this frittata airier. Cottage cheese will make it creamier, but if you prefer your frittata dairy-free, just omit. It will be delicious with or without.

Ingredients

2 tablespoons olive oil

6 button mushrooms, washed thoroughly and sliced

8–10 asparagus, washed thoroughly, woodsy ends snapped off, and cut into thirds

1/4 teaspoon kosher salt, divided

1/3 cup filtered water

2 cups egg whites

1/3 cup nonfat cottage cheese (optional)

Freshly ground black pepper, to taste

Cooking Instructions

1. Preheat the oven to 350 degrees.
2. Heat the oil in a nonstick, ovenproof pan until it begins to sizzle. Add the mushrooms and asparagus. Sauté on high heat for 2 to 3 minutes, stirring frequently to prevent sticking.
3. Season with half the salt. Add water and continue sautéing for another 2 to 3 minutes, until the vegetables soften and the liquids have evaporated. Turn off the heat. Spread the vegetable throughout the pan in a single layer.
4. In a large glass bowl, whisk the egg whites with remaining salt on medium high for 1 to 2 minutes until they become frothy and light.
5. Start reheating the pan with vegetables on medium high heat. Carefully pour the egg whites into the pan. Dot the frittata with dollops of cottage cheese, if using. Do not stir. Cover the pan and cook for 4 to 5 minutes until the edges of the frittata begin to bubble and solidify.
6. Remove the cover and place the pan in the center of the oven. Bake for 10 minutes. Turn on the broiler for another 2 minutes, allowing the frittata to char on top. Remove from the oven and allow to rest for 5 to 10 minutes before serving. The frittata will collapse a little and shrink away from the edges. Sprinkle with a few twists of freshly ground pepper, if desired. Serve hot, at room temperature, or cold. Refrigerate the leftovers, if any.

Prep and cooking time: 30 minutes
Serves 6

Smoked Salmon Burritos with an Herbed Egg Scramble and Avocado Stuffing

This no-fuss burrito for two is a carb-free indulgence, with smoked salmon serving as a wrap for herb-spiked scrambled eggs and smashed avocado that makes this dish smooth and exceptionally filling. If you are looking to break a 12- to 16-hour fast, this is a great choice that will satisfy a breakfast craving. On a plate, it looks like something you'd be served at a fine restaurant, but it takes less than 15 minutes to prepare from scratch and less than a minute to inhale if you're on the go.

Ingredients

4 slices of smoked salmon (approximately 2 ounces)

1/2 ripe Hass avocado

3 large eggs

2 tablespoons parsley, dill, basil leaves, or any combination of your favorite fresh herbs, finely chopped

Kosher salt, a dash plus 1/8 teaspoon for eggs

1/4 cup filtered water

Canola oil spray

Cooking Instructions

1. Arrange two slices of smoked salmon on each serving plate, making sure that the slices are overlapping by at least an inch. This is going to serve as the wrap for your scrambled eggs.
2. Using a fork, mash the avocado in a medium-size bowl with a dash of salt.
3. In another bowl, scramble the eggs, herbs, salt, and water.
4. Preheat a small nonstick pan. Spray with canola oil. Carefully pour the egg mixture into the pan and cook on medium low heat for 1 to 2 minutes until the mixture begins to stick to the bottom of the pan, forming a rim of cooked-through eggs around the edges. Using a thin metal spatula, carefully flip the eggs. Cook for another 1 to 2 minutes, until the eggs are cooked through.

5. Divide the eggs between two plates, placing them on top of the salmon slices, but leave enough room around the edge of the salmon to fold over the eggs in the next step.
6. Divide the mashed avocado between two plates, dolloping a spoonful on top of the eggs. Using your fingers, fold the salmon over the egg and avocado to make a pouch and carefully flip over so the salmon seam will be invisible. Serve immediately.

Prep and cooking time: 12–15 minutes
Serves 2

Deviled Tomatoes

In this twist on deviled eggs, the egg serves as a stuffing for a tomato shell, which makes for an attractive presentation and a nutritious breakfast or break-fast. You can make it a day in advance and refrigerate until ready to refuel your body.

Ingredients

3 hard-boiled eggs
1/4 teaspoon kosher salt
Freshly ground black pepper, to taste
2 tablespoons fresh dill leaves, chopped
2 sprigs of scallion, finely chopped, green and white parts separated
3 Roma tomatoes, halved lengthwise, seeds and flesh scooped out
1/8 teaspoon cayenne pepper

Cooking Instructions

1. Place the eggs in a small pan with enough water to cover them, bring the water to boil, reduce heat to low, and simmer, covered, for 5 to 7 minutes. Remove eggs from the water using a slotted spoon and place in a bowl filled with iced water. Allow the eggs to rest for 2 minutes in the water before removing the shell.
2. Using a fork, mash the eggs in a bowl until they reach a grainy consistency. Fold in salt, pepper, dill, and the white parts of the scallion.

3. Place the egg stuffing into the tomato shells. Dust each one with cayenne and top with the green parts of the scallions. Refrigerate if not eating right away.

Prep and cooking time: 15 minutes
Serves 6

Burger Bar, Three Ways

We've designed the turkey and lamb patties to be full of flavor but also suited for easy conversion to meatballs. We have a separate recipe for meatballs using ground beef or bison. (see page 186), but if you prefer lamb or turkey meatballs, the recipes for these burgers can be easily adjusted. All you need is a deep sauté pan and additional oil. Here are the basic conversion steps:

1. Once your turkey or lamb patty mixture is done, instead of dividing it into patties, roll it into 1½-inch meatballs.
2. Preheat the sauté pan with 2 tablespoons of olive oil.
3. When the oil begins to sizzle, carefully place the meatballs into the pan in batches of 10 to 15, depending on the size of your pan. Sear on high heat for 3 minutes per side. Try flipping the meatballs by rolling them around the pan and jiggling the handle. You can also flip the meatballs with a flat stainless-steel spatula. Don't press down on the meatballs with the spatula, as you will release the delicious juices.
4. Using a slotted spoon, remove the browned meatballs into a glass bowl and continue searing the remaining meatballs in batches, with additional oil as needed, until all meatballs are seared.
5. Turn off the heat. Carefully place all the browned meatballs back into the pan and cover for another 5 minutes to make sure they are cooked through.

The meatballs are delicious on a base of riced cauliflower, zoodles, or spaghetti squash. Coat the vegetable base with juices from the pan for extra flavor. Once cooked, the meatballs can be frozen for up to a month.

Bison Burger Patties

This recipe works with regular beef burgers, the tastiest of which has a protein-to-fat ratio of 80/20 percent, or an equal portion sirloin, chuck, and brisket combination. If you want a leaner but just as tasty option, then opt for ground bison, which is available in most chain grocery stores and sold in 12- to 16-ounce portions. Organic beef, if you can afford to splurge, is tastier, more environmentally sustainable, and better for you. (See "A Note on Cooking Oil Sprays" below.)

Ingredients

2 pounds bison or organic ground beef

2 tablespoons Worcestershire sauce

1 teaspoon kosher salt

2 teaspoons paprika

1 teaspoon ground celery seeds

1½ teaspoons garlic powder

1½ teaspoons onion powder

2 tablespoons olive oil (if you are using a stovetop grill)

Cooking Instructions (Stovetop Grill)

1. Using a wooden spoon or spatula, evenly combine all the ingredients except for the olive oil, but do not overmix.
2. Divide into 8 to 12 patties, depending on whether you want a substantial-size burger or a slider. Mold the patty into a smooth circle with a slight indentation in the middle, as it will expand vertically during the cooking process.
3. Preheat a nonstick grill pan on high. Using a silicone brush, spread olive oil in an even layer. (If your pan is on the small side and you need to cook the patties in batches, divide the olive oil accordingly. It doesn't have to be precise; just make sure there is enough oil to prevent the meat from sticking.) Cook on medium high heat 5 to 6 minutes per side. If you want your patties well done, after cooking on each side, turn off the heat, cover the pan, and let the patties rest for another 2 minutes.

Serve with the Bell Pepper and Onion Topping (p. 153) or Onions, Tomatoes, and Summer Squash Medley (p. 154).

Prep and cooking time: 25–30 minutes
Makes 8–12 patties, or 30–40 meatballs

A note on cooking sprays: There is some controversy about the use of chemicals in cooking sprays, but if that's your preferred method for grilling or sautéing, we recommend you use the organic variety. Cooking sprays are also more difficult to measure for portion control, which is the reason most of our recipes call for bottled olive oil. A good extra-virgin olive oil is also the most nutrient- and flavor-packed option.

Turkey Burger Patties

As far as taste and texture go, turkey meat is typically not the optimal choice for a tasty, juicy burger. Commercially made patties are delicious because they are filled with generous amounts of glutinous, sugary, and fatty ingredients that hold the meat together on the grill and give it the flavor and juices that it lacks naturally. This recipe is both healthier and tastier than anything you can get at the store or at a fast-food restaurant. Without bread crumbs the patty is a challenge to keep intact on an outdoor grill, so we recommend going stovetop on this one. Because these burgers incorporate dark meat for flavor, this recipe should be omitted from the first phase of the diet.

Ingredients

1/2 red onion
1 serrano or jalapeño pepper, stems removed and seeded for milder taste
1 tablespoon tomato paste
1 teaspoon kosher salt
1/4 teaspoon freshly ground black pepper
1/4 cup fresh parsley, with stems
1 tablespoon olive oil, more for pan searing
1 pound ground turkey breast
1 pound ground dark turkey meat
2 eggs

Cooking Instructions

1. In a food processor, combine all the ingredients except for the meat and eggs and pulse until this flavoring mixture reaches a smooth consistency.
2. In a large glass or stainless-steel bowl, combine the turkey meat with the flavoring mixture.
3. Add the eggs and mix, stirring with a wooden spoon until the meat is thoroughly incorporated. Don't overmix. Cover with plastic wrap and refrigerate for at least an hour.
4. To cook, divide the meat into 8 to 12 patties, depending on whether you want substantial-size burgers or sliders.
5. Preheat a nonstick stovetop grill. Brush with olive oil, 1 tablespoon at a time if you are grilling in batches. Add the patties to the pan and cook on medium high heat, 5 minutes per side. Be careful when turning the patties over, as they are prone to falling apart. Top with Onions, Tomatoes, and Summer Squash Medley (p. 154), Red Pepper Tahini Spread (p. 156), or both. Serve immediately.

Prep and cooking time: 35–45 minutes
Makes 8–12 patties, or 30–40 meatballs

Lamb Burgers

If you are doing a burger bar and would like to offer a more gourmet option, include a lamb patty in your offerings, which will give your spread a touch of Mediterranean flair. (If you like the taste of Greek gyro, you will love the taste of lamb burger!) Some people don't like the gaminess of lamb, which is why we mix it with ground sirloin beef for a hint of familiar flavor. A touch of baking soda will make the patty especially plump, and a sprinkle of paprika and sumac (a Mediterranean, slightly acidic spice) will give it a deep garnet color. A lamb burger pairs ideally with a tahini-based condiment, such as Red Pepper Tahini Spread (p. 156) or our Basic Tahini Sauce (p. 155). But for a truly low-maintenance experience, nothing pairs better with a juicy lamb burger than a slice of a naturally sweet beefsteak tomato and a red onion.

Ingredients

3 sprigs of scallion, white and green parts, chopped

Fresh mint, leaves of 1/2 bunch, or 1/4 cup

Cilantro, leaves of 1/2 bunch, or 1/4 cup

1 tablespoon olive oil, more if you are cooking the burgers on the stovetop

1 pound ground lamb

1/2 pound ground beef

1/8 teaspoon baking soda

1/2 teaspoon kosher salt

1 tablespoon paprika

2 teaspoons sumac*

1 tablespoon za'atar*

1 tablespoon harissa sauce*

1 egg

Cooking Instructions

1. In a blender, pulse scallions, mint, cilantro, and olive oil until the mixture reaches a pasty consistency.
2. In a large glass bowl, combine the rest of the ingredients and mix thoroughly using a wooden spoon. Do not overmix. Cover with plastic wrap and refrigerate until you are ready to grill, but for at least 1 hour.
3. Make the patties of your desired size (should make 6 to 8 patties).
4. To prepare on a stovetop grill, heat the grill on medium high and brush the pan with olive oil or cooking spray. For a medium to well-done burger, cook 3 to 4 minutes per side. Turn off the heat and keep

---

*You can buy za'atar, sumac, and harissa sauce at well-stocked specialty grocers such as Whole Foods or on Amazon, although more and more stores carry them in their Middle Eastern sections. If you prefer to use the ingredients already in your pantry, you can substitute a mix of ground cumin seeds, sesame seeds, and ground thyme (1 teaspoon of each) for the za'atar, a zest of one lemon for the sumac, and any bottle of hot pepper sauce for the harissa.

the patties in the pan, covered, for another 2 to 3 minutes. Lamb burgers tend to burn more on the stovetop, so keep an eye on them as you cook and keep your pan generously oiled.

Prep and cooking time: 35–45 minutes
Makes 6–8 burger patties, or 30–40 meatballs

Burger Toppings

Bell Pepper and Onion Topping for Bison/Beef Burgers

This vitamin-rich, colorful vegetable medley retains its crunch while infusing your meals with complex flavor. It is a great side dish for any grilled red meat or poultry, but its smokiness makes it a particularly good pairing with an old-fashioned beef burger. A splash of mescal, if you have it, creates another layer of the outdoor experience. Don't sweat it if you have only one variety of bell pepper on hand. Color makes the dish more attractive, but it doesn't change the taste. If you don't want this topping to be too spicy, omit the serrano pepper. For best results, sauté the vegetables separately and combine in a serving dish.

Ingredients

1 tablespoon olive oil, divided
1/2 teaspoon kosher salt, divided
1/2 red onion, sliced thinly into half-moon shape
1 poblano pepper, stemmed and seeded, cut into strips
1 red bell pepper, stemmed and seeded, cut into strips
1 orange bell pepper, stemmed and seeded, cut into strips
1 serrano pepper, stem removed (optional)
Freshly ground black pepper, to taste
1 teaspoon ancho chili powder
2 teaspoons mescal (optional)
1 tablespoon sherry vinegar
Fresh thyme leaves from 1 sprig, more if you want to create a woodsier aroma

Cooking Instructions

1. Preheat half the olive oil on high heat in a nonstick pan. Sauté the onions with half the salt, stirring frequently to prevent burning, for about 5 minutes. If the onions start to burn, add a splash of water, 1 tablespoon at a time. Ideally, the onions should be cooked but retain a slight crunch. Remove the onions from the pan and place in a storage or serving container.
2. Add the rest of the oil to the pan. When it starts to sizzle, add the peppers. Cook for 3 to 5 minutes, stirring infrequently, to allow the peppers to char. Add remaining salt and spices and mix thoroughly. Add mescal, if using, stirring until the alcohol evaporates. Add vinegar and stir for another 1 to 2 minute until peppers caramelize.
3. Combine the peppers with the onions and sprinkle with fresh thyme. Serve at room temperature.

Prep and cooking time: 20–25 minutes
Serves 8–12 as a topping, 6 as a side dish

Onion, Tomato, and Summer Squash Medley (a side dish or topping for bison/beef burgers)

This raw vegetable topping also doubles nicely as a side salad with red meat, poultry, or fish. Summer squash (more commonly known as zucchini) and beefsteak tomatoes are a heavenly mix and offer a nice, more gourmet variation on the standard onion and tomato topping for burgers. A couple notes on this recipe: only the onions and squash should be pickled (the pickling will be mild given the relatively short amount of time); beefsteak tomatoes are naturally sweet so the vinegar and salt, which tend to draw the natural juices out, are best added to tomatoes right before serving. If you don't have access to beefsteak tomatoes, a smaller but sturdy variety will do. A teaspoon of honey is optional; you will not taste the sweetness, but it will bring out the flavors of the onions and squash. To serve this topping as a salad, sprinkle it with fresh summer herbs, like basil leaves or cilantro.

Ingredients

1 large Vidalia or other sweet white onion, sliced into thin half-moons
1 garlic clove, crushed
1/2 teaspoon crushed pepper flakes, more, if you want the veggies spicier
1/4 teaspoon kosher salt
1 teaspoon honey (optional)
1 green zucchini, skin on, washed thoroughly and sliced into thin ovals*
1 yellow zucchini, washed thoroughly and sliced into thin ovals*
1/4 cup white wine vinegar
1 beefsteak tomato or 6 smaller tomatoes, sliced into thick circles

Cooking Instructions

1. Combine all the ingredients except the tomatoes and refrigerate. Allow to pickle for at least 2 hours before serving.
2. Drain the zucchini and onions and discard the garlic clove. Place in a shallow bowl in a single layer. Top with tomatoes right before serving. Drizzle with more salt, vinegar, and olive oil if desired.

Prep and cooking time: 15 minutes, more for pickling
Serves 8–12 as burger topping, 6 as a side dish salad

Basic Tahini Sauce

You've tasted this sauce if you've ever been to a Greek or Middle Eastern restaurant, where it is usually served as a condiment for gyros. It also works as a base for a salad dressing and homemade hummus, for the non-dieters in your family. If you want to take it up a notch, you can add a clove of crushed garlic, a pinch of red pepper, or a cluster of any soft leafy fresh herb from your garden.

Ingredients

1/3 cup tahini paste
1/3 cup ice-cold water
A pinch of kosher salt
Juice of 1 lemon

*Some varieties of green and yellow zucchini can have large seeds, which don't add flavor but can add an unpleasant texture. Feel free to scoop out the seeds with a serrated spoon (like a grapefruit spoon) prior to slicing.

Cooking Instructions

1. In a medium-size glass or stainless-steel bowl, vigorously whisk the tahini paste with water. It will resist at first, but you'll know you've beaten it down when it turns silky smooth.
2. Add the rest of the ingredients and whisk some more. Refrigerate until ready to use. It will thicken over time, but you can dilute it to desired consistency with more icy water or lemon juice if desired.

Prep and cooking time: 10 minutes
Makes 2/3 cup

Red Pepper Tahini Spread for Turkey Burgers

This naturally sweet and exotic condiment will make you forget ketchup on your burgers. It can also stand in for mayo in sandwiches and provides a reliable sauce for any meat or poultry dish. In a pinch, it can be served as a basic vegetable dip. You can eliminate most of the cooking and prep time by using peeled, jarred peppers. As always, food made from scratch is healthier because it has less added sugar and fat. But if you are in a hurry, use the prepared stuff. Just make sure to rinse the peppers to remove all the acid and chemical toxins in the preservatives.

Ingredients

3 red bell peppers (if using fresh)

1/3 cup tahini paste

1/3 cup filtered ice-cold water

1 teaspoon salt

Juice of 1½ lemons

1 serrano or jalapeño pepper, stemmed and seeded if the latter

1/3 cup fresh cilantro leaves, with stems

Cooking Instructions

1. Preheat the oven to 400 degrees. Line a baking sheet with aluminum foil or parchment paper and place whole bell peppers on top. Roast for 45 minutes, turning the peppers with silicone tongs (metal tongs can puncture the pepper) every 15 minutes.

2. While the bell peppers are roasting, prepare the tahini base. Combine the paste with water, salt, and lemon juice, whisking vigorously until the paste thins out to a consistency of glue.
3. Remove the peppers from the oven and, using silicone tongs, place in paper bags, gently sealing them. (This will allow the skin to come off effortlessly.) Allow to cool completely.
4. Clean the peppers by removing the skin, stems, and seeds but retaining the juices.
5. Place bell peppers and juices in the food processor. Add the prepared tahini mix, serrano or jalapeño peppers, and cilantro and blend until smooth.
6. Place in a sealed container and refrigerate for at least 2 hours prior to serving so the flavors can deepen and the mixture thicken. Serve cold or at room temperature.

Prep and cooking time: 1 hour
Serves 8–12

Taco Bar, Three Ways

Taco Fillings

Tri Tip Steak

Tri Tip Steak, so popular in California, is known in other parts of the country as top sirloin. It is a juicy, delicious cut of beef that's perfect for grilling and taco fillings, and can be marinated up to 2 days in advance. This basic go-to recipe works for the classic soft or hard tortilla shells. Unless it's your Cheat Meal, however, you'll want to use radicchio, endive, or Boston lettuce leaves instead. Leftover steak can be used with Cauliflower "Rice," Chinese Style (p. 179) or as a salad topping.

Ingredients

1 teaspoon kosher salt

1½ teaspoons paprika

Freshly ground black pepper, to taste

1/2 teaspoon chipotle powder

Juice of 1 lime

2 tablespoons olive oil

1½ pounds top sirloin

Cooking Instructions

1. Make the marinade by mixing spices with the lime juice and olive oil. Whisk thoroughly and massage into the beef. Marinate, refrigerated, for at least 8 hours. The longer it sits, the better it will taste.
2. To prepare on the stovetop, preheat the oven to 350 degrees. In an ovenproof grill pan, brown the meat on both sides, 5 to 7 minutes each.
3. Move the pan into the oven and bake for another 10 minutes for medium rare, 12 to 15 minutes for medium or well done. Allow to rest for 5 to 10 minutes before slicing. Cut the meat against the grain into thin slices.
4. For tacos, serve in a tortilla or lettuce shell, with avocado slices or guacamole and your choice of homemade salsa.

Prep and cooking time: 35–40 minutes, plus marinating time
Serves 12 as part of a taco bar, 6 for a standard meal

Grilled Chicken Breasts

These chicken breasts can be served in slices at your taco bar or as two whole pieces on a more elegant dinner plate. Please note cooking time may vary based upon thickness of chicken breasts used.

Ingredients

1/2 teaspoon chipotle powder

1/2 teaspoon Mexican oregano

1/2 teaspoon garlic powder

1 teaspoon ground coriander

1 tablespoon olive oil

2 boneless chicken breasts

Spray canola or olive oil

Cooking Instructions

1. To make the marinade, whisk the first five ingredients in a small bowl. Coat the chicken breasts and refrigerate for at least 2 hours before cooking.
2. Preheat a grill pan on high heat. Spray or brush lightly with oil (watch splatters), and place the chicken on the pan, reducing heat to medium high. Cook from 4–6 minutes on each side.
3. Turn off the heat and cover the pan for another 3 to 4 minutes before serving. For a taco bar, slice into strips of your desired thickness.
4. Wrap in a tortilla (for non-dieters) or a lettuce leaf with your choice of Tomatillo Salsa (p. 160) or Roasted Tomato Salsa (p. 161) and avocado slices or Basic Guacamole (p. 162). Serve immediately.

Prep and cooking time: 12–15 minutes, plus marinating time
Serves 6 as part of larger taco bar, 2 for traditional meal

Easy Shrimp Filling for Tacos, Shrimp Cocktail, or Salad Toppings

The best way to make shrimp for all occasions came from the great Ina Garten, who gave these simple instructions: Preheat the oven to 400 degrees, put the shrimp on a lined baking sheet, and bake for exactly 6 minutes. The texture will be perfect—never over or undercooked, which is a common problem with shrimp. How you spice the shrimp is up to you, but this version tastes great when served warm, at room temperature, or cold. In a taco bar, you can use an endive leaf instead of a tortilla and serve the shrimp with Tomatillo Salsa (p. 160) or Roasted Tomato Salsa (p. 161) and Basic Guacamole (p. 162). If you want to serve this as a shrimp cocktail, do so with our Quick Romesco Sauce (p. 196).

Ingredients

1 pound raw shrimp, peeled and deveined, tails off (unless you are using for cocktail, in which case leave the tail on for easy pick-up with fingers)

2 tablespoons Worcestershire sauce

1/4 teaspoon kosher salt

Freshly ground black pepper, to taste

Cooking Instructions

1. Preheat the oven to 400 degrees.
2. Place the shrimp in a large bowl and carefully pat dry with paper towel to remove excess moisture. Season with Worcestershire sauce, salt, and pepper.
3. Line a baking sheet with aluminum foil or parchment paper. Place the shrimp in a single layer and bake for exactly 6 minutes. Remove from the oven and serve immediately or at room temperature. Refrigerate for later use.

Prep and cooking time: 10–12 minutes
Serves 6 in a taco bar, as an appetizer, or a salad topping

Taco Toppings

Tomatillo Salsa

Tomatillos are a seasonal fruit (in peak during late summer and early fall) and are often mistaken for green tomatoes. While tomato and tomatillo plants are related, they are not interchangeable. A staple of Mexican and Guatemalan cuisine, the tomatillo is the main ingredient in green salsas. In grocery stores they can be found in the vegetable aisle and are sold in husks, which have to be removed prior to cooking. Tomatillos offer a distinctly tart bite to any taco and make a colorful sauce for seafood, poultry, pork, and fish. If you are making tomatillo sauce for tacos, serve it alongside Roasted Tomato Salsa (p. 161). Homemade salsas are a breeze to make and are always a healthier alternative to the commercial jarred varieties. They can be made a day in advance and refrigerated up to a week.

Ingredients

1/2 garlic bulb

2 tablespoons olive oil, divided

Kosher salt, a dash for the garlic plus one 1 teaspoon

5 tomatillos, husks removed and washed thoroughly

1 poblano pepper

3 sprigs of green onion

1/2 cup fresh cilantro leaves

Juice of 1/2 lime

Cooking Instructions

1. Preheat the oven to 400 degrees. Line a baking sheet with aluminum foil or parchment paper. Carefully cut a garlic bulb in half horizontally. Brush the half you are using with olive oil, sprinkle with salt, and wrap in foil. Place the half garlic bulb along with the tomatillos and poblano pepper on the lined baking sheet and roast for 40 to 45 minutes, turning the vegetables, if they start burning, every 20 minutes.
2. Allow the vegetables to cool to room temperature. Remove the stem and seeds from the poblano pepper. Squeeze the garlic from its shell into a small bowl.
3. Place the tomatillos, poblano pepper, and garlic into a large food processor. Add green onions, cilantro, and lime juice. Pulse, adding the remaining olive oil in a thin stream, until it reaches a desired consistency. Refrigerate for at least an hour before serving.

Prep and cooking time: 1 hour
Makes 1½ to 2 cups

Roasted Tomato Salsa

A staple condiment at any taco bar, Roasted Tomato Salsa is much more delicious homemade than a jarred, store-bought one, which comes packaged with preservatives none of us can pronounce. For this recipe, any small, juicy tomato will do. We recommend roasting tomatoes in a glass casserole to capture the juices. If you want a milder salsa, remove the stem and seeds from the jalapeño before roasting.

Ingredients

10 ounces of juicy tomatoes (beefsteak, Holland, cherry, heirloom, or whatever is in season)

1/2 garlic bulb

1 jalapeño pepper

1/2 small or 1/4 large red onion

2 tablespoons olive oil

1/2 teaspoon Mexican oregano

1/2 teaspoon chipotle powder

1/2 teaspoon kosher salt

3 sprigs of savory (optional)

Juice of 1/2 lime

1/2 cup fresh cilantro leaves

Cooking Instructions

1. Preheat the oven to 400 degrees. Place the tomatoes, garlic bulb (cut-side down), jalapeño pepper, and onion in a glass casserole glass. Drizzle with olive oil and sprinkle with oregano, chipotle powder, salt, and savory, if using. Roast for 30 to 35 minutes, until the tomatoes start blistering. Remove from the oven and allow the ingredients to cool to room temperature.
2. Squeeze the garlic out of the shell and into a food processor. If you roasted the entire jalapeño, remove the stem.
3. Place the roasted ingredients and the released juices into the food processor. Add lime juice and cilantro. Pulse until the salsa reaches your desired consistency.

Prep and cooking time: 45 minutes, more for cooling
Makes 1 cup; refrigerate leftovers for up to 1 week

Basic Guacamole

There are as many recipes for guacamole as there are families in Mexico and California, but this one is so easy you will memorize it after making it just once. Serve it as a dip, a topping, a spread, or, if you are like me, as a meal! If you are using it for a taco bar or serving it at a party, sprinkle with citric acid so the green flesh of the avocado doesn't turn brown. A large mortar and pestle is optional when making guacamole, but it will make the guacamole more aromatic and smoother than the more conventional approach of mashing it with a fork.

Ingredients

3 plum tomatoes, core and seeds removed, chopped

1 large or 2 small shallots, peeled and diced

1 jalapeño pepper, stem and seeds removed for milder flavor, and chopped

1 teaspoon kosher salt

1/2 cup fresh cilantro leaves, chopped

Juice of 1 lime

Flesh of 2 ripe Haas avocadoes

1/8 teaspoon citric acid (optional)

Cooking Instructions

1. Place all the ingredients except the avocados in a mortar and crush with a pestle to release their juices and fragrances.
2. Add the flesh of the avocados and mash some more until the mixture reaches your desired consistency.
3. Adjust seasoning, sprinkle on citric acid (if using), cover with plastic wrap, and refrigerate until ready to serve.

Prep and cooking time: 15 minutes
Serves 6

Pizza Night, Three Ways

Our Cauliflower Pizza Crust forms the base for the three delicious pizzas that follow.

Cauliflower Pizza Crust (Phase 2 only)

Gluten intolerance was the necessity behind this great culinary invention, but even those who don't suffer from this food sensitivity can enjoy a wheat-free, nutrient rich alternative to conventionally carb-loaded crust. Plus, there is an extra benefit of enjoying a pizza that is filling with just a single slice. Because cauliflower, almonds, and other ingredients in the crust combine to offer a healthy dose of fiber, this pizza will digest slowly, allowing for a more relaxed fasting interval. And there are other benefits for making the crust at home: a prepared 6-inch cauliflower crust sold frozen at a gourmet grocery store can set you back $7 to $10, and it can still be loaded with gluten-free but caloric flour. A homemade cauliflower crust can be made for a fraction of the cost and the batter frozen for future use. Bake it Roman style on a large rectangular baking sheet, or divide into two round pizza pans.

Ingredients

Florets of 1 medium head of cauliflower, trimmed and washed

2 teaspoons kosher salt for riced cauliflower, plus 1/2 teaspoon for the dry ingredients

2 cups almond flour, more for dusting the baking sheet

1/4 teaspoon freshly ground black pepper

1/4 teaspoon garlic powder

1/4 teaspoon dry basil or parsley

2 tablespoons ground Parmesan cheese

2 large eggs

2 teaspoons olive oil

Cooking Instructions

1. In a large food processor, pulse the cauliflower florets in batches until they reach grain-like consistency. It should yield approximately 3 cups.
2. Place the riced cauliflower into a glass bowl and microwave for 4 minutes, 2 minutes at a time. In between, stir to make sure it is cooking evenly.
3. In a fine-meshed strainer large enough to hold all the riced cauliflower, rinse with cold water. Place over a bowl and add salt. Allow the cauliflower to drain for 10 to 12 minutes, squeezing out the water with your hands aggressively. The volume should reduce by at least half.*
4. While the cauliflower is draining, prepare the dry ingredients by whisking the almond flour with the salt, pepper, garlic powder, basil or parsley, and Parmesan cheese.

---

*If you are squeamish about using your hands to squeeze the water out of the steamed cauliflower, then place the cauliflower in a cheesecloth, tie the top in a knot, and squeeze the liquids out.

5. Add the cauliflower and eggs to the dry ingredients. Fold carefully until the mixture forms into a solid batter.
6. Form the batter into a circular sphere and place in a plastic wrap. Freeze for 1/2 to 1 hour.
7. Preheat the oven to 425 degrees.
8. Line a baking sheet with parchment paper, brush with olive oil, and dust with 1 to 2 tablespoons of almond flour.
9. Carefully remove the batter from the freezer and place in the middle of the baking sheet. Spread it over the sheet with a rolling pin and finish filling it manually with your hands. Remember that there is no gluten in this crust, so it doesn't coalesce naturally. But not to worry—it will bake into a smooth, even crust.
10. Bake for 20 to 25 minutes until the crust is dry at the center and the edges begin to crust. Remove from the oven and bring to room temperature. Proceed to create a pizza with the toppings of your choice.

Prep and cooking time: 1 hour 45 minutes
Serves 8–10

The Siesta Salad Pizza

The possibilities for "salad pizza" are endless. Feel free to improvise with your favorite toppings from the food lists, but keep a few tips in mind: Opt for a sturdier green leaf, like an arugula, to keep the pizza from getting soggy. Don't overdress the vegetables, and use a condiment like an olive or sundried tomato tapenade or a pesto as an adhesive between the pizza crust and toppings. Whatever vegetable toppings you choose, make sure you dress them in a bowl before building the layers on the crust; this will keep the salad lighter and fluffier and the crust crisp. For easier serving, cut the crust into slices prior to assembling the pizza. And lastly, avocado oil gives all salad dressings a slightly floral scent but if you don't have it, substitute with olive oil, preferably unfiltered, which is more pure and intense. To save time, prepare the topping while the crust bakes.

Ingredients

9- to 12-inch Cauliflower Pizza Crust, homemade (p. 163) or store bought

1/4 teaspoon kosher salt

1 tablespoon white wine vinegar

2 tablespoons olive oil

1 tablespoon avocado oil

3 cups wild baby arugula

2/3 cup cherry tomatoes, sliced in halves

1/3 cup pitted Niçoise olives, chopped

2 tablespoons sundried tomato tapenade

3 ounces San Danielle prosciutto, excess fat removed, sliced into thin strips

4 ounces goat cheese

Cooking Instructions

1. Bake the pizza crust (p. 164); if store bought, bake according to package instructions.
2. In a large bowl, prepare the dressing by diluting salt in the vinegar and whisking in the oils in a thin stream until fully emulsified.
3. Place the arugula, cherry tomatoes, and olives into the bowl and, using tongs or salad spoons, coat with the dressing from the bottom of the bowl up. (This bottom-to-top technique allows for a fluffier salad.)
4. Place the tapenade in the center of the crust and, using the back of a spoon, spread it evenly to coat approximately 3/4 of the crust sphere. Lightly preslice the crust.
5. Using tongs, place the dressed salad on top of the crust. Place the prosciutto strips and small dollops of goat cheese, spreading them at desired intervals throughout the salad. To prevent the salad from spilling, serve individual portions using a wide stainless-steel spatula.

Prep and cooking time: 20 minutes for the salad, more for baking the crust

Serves 4

The "Southwestern Delight" Salad Pizza

This pizza for the grown-up palate offers up a variety of textures—creamy (avocado), crunchy (pepitas), and earthy (sprouts) and makes for a gourmet feast for the health and weight conscious. Just like all our cauliflower crust pizzas, it is a complete, satisfying meal on a dainty plate.

Ingredients

9- to 12-inch Cauliflower Pizza Crust, homemade (p. 163) or store bought

1 tablespoon pepitas

1/4 teaspoon kosher salt

1 tablespoon sherry vinegar

1 tablespoon avocado oil

2 tablespoons extra-virgin olive oil

2 cups wild baby arugula

1 cup radish sprouts

2/3 cup shredded carrot

3 radishes, sliced

2 tablespoons pesto sauce

1 avocado, pitted and flesh sliced into thin strips

Juice of 1/2 lime

1 teaspoon Spike seasoning

Cooking Instructions

1. Bake the pizza crust (p. 164); if store bought, bake according to package instructions.
2. In a preheated nonstick pan, toast pepitas for 30 to 60 seconds, removing from heat as soon as the seeds begin to brown. Be careful not to burn them, which happens quickly. Place the seeds in a separate bowl and allow to cool completely.
3. In a bowl big enough to hold the salad ingredients, prepare the dressing by diluting salt in the vinegar and whisking in the oils in a steady, thin stream until fully emulsified.

4. To the salad dressing add arugula, sprouts, carrot, radishes, and pepitas. Using salad spoons or tongs, coat the salad ingredients with the dressing from bottom up until fully integrated.
5. Using the back of a serving spoon, spread the pesto onto the baked crust from the center in an even layer, covering approximately 3/4 of the crust sphere. Lightly preslice the crust.
6. Using tongs, carefully place dressed salad on top of the crust. Scatter the avocado slices, sprinkle with lime juice, and top with Spike. Serve immediately.

Prep and cooking time: 20 minutes, plus baking of the crust
Serves 4–6

Healthy Hawaiian Pizza

If you like your pizza sweet and savory, you'll love this dish. To maintain balance between these two flavors, we recommend cutting the bacon and the pineapple into bite-size pieces and sautéing them prior to finishing the pizza in the oven. This will allow the sugar in the pineapple to caramelize and the bacon to crisp. And because both the pineapple and bacon bits will be small, the savory/sweet sensation will taste more unified. Place the pizza under the broiler at the end of the baking process to allow the cheesy gooeyness to bubble over. Serve this pizza piping hot.

Ingredients

12-inch Cauliflower Pizza Crust, homemade (p. 163) or store bought

1 tablespoon olive oil

4 ounces Canadian bacon, cubed

3 ounces pineapple chunks, cubed

1/2 cup store-bought pizza sauce

1 cup shredded cheese (combination of fontina, white cheddar, and Parmesan)

4 ounces fresh mozzarella, sliced in circles

2 sprigs of scallion, white and green parts, chopped

Cooking Instructions

1. Bake the crust (p. 164); if store bought, bake according to package instructions. As soon as the crust is baked and removed from oven, preheat it to 500 degrees.
2. Heat the oil in a nonstick pan and sauté the bacon for 60 to 90 seconds until the edges begin to brown. Using a slotted spoon, remove to a bowl or plate lined with a paper towel to absorb excess grease.
3. In the same pan, sauté pineapple chunks for another 60 to 90 seconds until the edges of the pineapple begin to brown. Add to the bowl with bacon.
4. Prepare the baked crust. Using the back of a spoon, spread the pizza sauce from the center in widening circles until all but the edge of the crust is coated.
5. Spread the cheese evenly over the crust. Top with a layer of mozzarella slices, followed by a layer of bacon and pineapple, spacing them evenly throughout the crust.
6. Return the pizza to the oven and bake for 12 minutes. Turn on the broiler and broil for another 2 minutes. Remove from the oven, sprinkle with scallions, slice into serving pieces, and serve immediately.

Prep and cooking time: 20–25 minutes, more for baking the pizza crust
Serves 4–6

Superstar Veggie Dishes

String Bean, Tomato, and Turkey Bacon Medley (side or main dish)

This side dish is meaty enough to be a main course for someone looking to refuel after a long fast. The challenge in this dish is to keep the string beans crispy and brightly colored. As a side dish, it goes well with fish, meat, or poultry.

Ingredients

3 tablespoons olive oil, divided into thirds

10 ounces turkey bacon, cut into small pieces (the smaller, the better)

1 pound fresh string beans (green, yellow, or combination), ends trimmed and cut in thirds

1 teaspoon kosher salt

10 ounces grape tomatoes

1 garlic clove, crushed

1 teaspoon red pepper flakes

1 cluster of scallions, white and green parts, chopped

1/4 cup capers, chopped

Cooking Instructions

1. Preheat a nonstick pan and brush it with 1/3 of the oil. Add the bacon and cook until it reaches desired crispiness, approximately 7 to 10 minutes. Remove from pan into a glass bowl lined with a paper towel to absorb excess grease.
2. Brush the pan with another 1/3 of the olive oil and add the string beans. Cook, stirring frequently, for 4 to 5 minutes. Add salt. Remove from pan into the bowl with bacon.
3. Brush pan with the final third of the olive oil and add tomatoes, garlic clove, red pepper flakes, scallions, onions, and capers. Cook until the tomatoes blister, about 3 to 5 minutes. Combine thoroughly with string bean and bacon mixture. Serve at room temperature.

Prep and cooking time: 30–35 minutes
Serves 12 as a side dish, 6 as a main course

Roasted Tomato, Wilted Leafy Greens, and Sautéed Mushroom Platter

This back to basics, nutrient-dense assortment of lightly cooked vegetables tastes as scrumptious as it looks on a plate and makes a perfect side dish for a frittata breakfast, lunch, or dinner. Or, double the portion and eat it as a full meal! Use your favorite sturdy green-leaf vegetable—kale, Swiss chard, escarole, dandelion greens, and baby spinach work best—but remember that sturdier leaf requires a little more time and a splash of water to wilt. For this reason, I also recommend that if you are using baby spinach, don't mix it with the other greens, as it has a different texture when cooked. For tastiest results and most attractive presentation, cook the greens and mushrooms separately, resisting the temptation to save time by cooking them together. The elongated Roma tomatoes, which are at their best in summer, are especially good for roasting because of their low water content. Prepare and serve these vegetables on a single platter or separately, if you wish.

For the Roasted Tomatoes:

Ingredients

1 teaspoon olive oil

5 Roma tomatoes, cut in half vertically

1/8 teaspoon kosher salt

Freshly ground black pepper, to taste

Cooking Instructions

1. Preheat the oven to 400 degrees. Line a baking sheet with aluminum foil or parchment paper and brush with olive oil.
2. Season the tomatoes with salt and pepper and place on the baking sheet cut-side down.
3. Roast 7 minutes on one side and flip over using a stainless-steel spatula. Roast for another 7 to 10 minutes, until the tomatoes soften but don't lose their shape. Remove from the oven and allow to cool completely.

For the Mushrooms:

Ingredients

1 teaspoon olive oil

8 ounces baby portabella mushrooms, cleaned with a wet paper towel to remove grime and quartered

1/8 teaspoon kosher salt

Freshly ground black pepper, to taste

Leaves of fresh lemon thyme, 6 sprigs

1 tablespoon fresh parsley leaves

1 tablespoon fresh dill leaves

Cooking Instructions

1. Preheat a nonstick pan brushed with oil on medium high heat.
2. Add the mushrooms, salt, and pepper and sauté, turning periodically, for 10 minutes, turning the heat down to medium when the mushrooms begin to char. Sprinkle with water to loosen the mushrooms if they stick to the bottom of the pan.
3. When the mushrooms start to release moisture, about 5 minutes into the sauté process, add the herbs.
4. Remove from pan and wipe it clean.

For the Wilted Greens:

Ingredients

2 teaspoons olive oil

8 ounces kale, Swiss chard, dandelion greens, or a combination, stems removed and roughly chopped (double the portion if you are using baby spinach)

1/8 teaspoon kosher salt

2 garlic cloves, peeled and smashed

1/8 teaspoon red pepper flakes

Cooking Instructions

1. Preheat the oil in the pan you used for the mushrooms.
2. Add the greens and salt and stir.
3. When the greens start to wilt, add garlic cloves and red pepper flakes and sauté for 5 to 7 minutes, until they release their juices and those juices have evaporated. The volume of greens should reduce dramatically as they sauté, to about 1/3 the original amount. They are ready when they have completely wilted.

Serve the roasted tomatoes, leafy greens, and mushrooms at room temperature on a platter, either separately or stacked. If you stack the vegetables, place the greens at the bottom, the mushrooms in the middle, and tomatoes on top. Sprinkle with more fresh herbs if desired.

Prep and cooking time: 20–25 minutes for each vegetable
Serves 6

Roasted Fennel, Brussels Sprouts, and Butternut Squash*

This tasty comfort food side dish is perfect with fish or poultry, but it is sturdy enough to be a filling vegan meal. Roast the vegetables on separate baking sheets because the fennel cooks and burns faster than the butternut squash.

For the Fennel:

The bright green fennel fronds make the dish colorful and aromatic enough for any family-style feast, whether it's a casual or elegant meal. Don't let the fennel linger prior to roasting; it tends to brown. If you think it will take you a while to get it into the oven, sprinkle with lemon juice.

Ingredients

4 fennel bulbs, fibrous outer layers and core removed, and quartered (reserve stalks for soups and broths, and reserve fronds, chopped, for serving)

1 tablespoon olive oil

1/2 teaspoon kosher salt

Freshly ground black pepper, to taste

3 leaves fresh sage, finely chopped, or 1/4 teaspoon dry sage

3 sprigs of fresh rosemary leaves, finely chopped, or 1/4 teaspoon dry rosemary leaves

3 sprigs of fresh thyme, or 1/4 teaspoon dry thyme

Juice of 1/2 lemon

---

*Omit butternut squash in Phase 1.

Cooking Instructions

1. Preheat the oven to 450 degrees. Line the baking sheet with aluminum foil.
2. Place the fennel on the baking sheet in a single layer, brush with oil, and sprinkle with spices and herbs (except the fennel fronds).
3. Roast for 15 minutes and turn to other side using tongs or a stainless-steel spatula. Roast for another 10 minutes, until the fennel is fork tender. Remove from the oven, sprinkle with lemon juice and 1/2 of fennel fronds, and fold the edges of the foil, making a pouch that will allow the fennel to steam to perfection and the aromatic herbs and spices to meld for another 10 minutes.

Prep and cooking time: 45 minutes
Serves 4–6

For the Brussels Sprouts:

Ingredients

2 pounds Brussels sprouts, core trimmed and outer leaves removed

2 teaspoons olive oil

1/4 teaspoon kosher salt

Freshly ground black pepper, to taste

Cooking Instructions

1. Preheat the oven to 375 degrees. Line a baking sheet with aluminum foil or parchment paper.
2. Coat the Brussels sprouts with olive oil and sprinkle with salt and pepper by tossing in a bowl.
3. Scatter around the baking sheet in a single layer and roast for 45 minutes, flipping them every 15 minutes to make sure they don't burn and are cooked through evenly. Remove from the oven. Serve hot, at room temperature, or cold, as a side dish or as a vegetarian meal along with Wilted Leafy Greens (p. 170) and/or Roasted Butternut Squash (p. 175).

Prep and cooking time: 1 to 1½ hours
Serves 6–8

For the Butternut Squash:

When buying butternut squash, look for one that has the most elongated stem. These are easier to cube than the seeded bulb, which doesn't always accommodate a pairing knife. (You can save the tops for soup; if soup is not on the menu, just toss them in the compost bin.)

Ingredients

2 medium or 1 large butternut squash, stem peeled with a sharp pairing knife, and cubed

Cooking spray (olive oil or canola)

1 tablespoon olive oil

1/2 teaspoon kosher salt

Freshly ground black pepper, to taste

1/2 teaspoon dry basil

1/2 teaspoon celery seeds

Juice of 1/2 lemon

Fresh nutmeg nut, grated to taste

Cooking Instructions

1. Preheat the oven to 450 degrees. Line a baking sheet with aluminum foil and spray with oil.
2. Line up the cubed butternut squash in a single layer. Brush with olive oil and sprinkle with salt, pepper, basil, and celery seed. Roast for 10 minutes and turn over, roasting on the other side for another 10 to 15 minutes until the butternut squash is fork tender. Remove from the oven. Sprinkle with lemon juice and dust with nutmeg.
3. Fold the edges of the foil to create a pouch, allowing the squash to steam for another 10 minutes.
4. Combine butternut squash and fennel in a single dish and serve at room temperature or slightly warmed, with a sprinkle of remaining fennel fronds on top.

Prep and cooking time: 45 minutes
Serves 4–6

Pan-Seared Asparagus

Asparagus pairs with Petite Filet Mignon (p. 183) like peaches with cream or chocolate with marshmallows. But you can also eat asparagus with any other meat or vegetable, or even serve it by itself. Remember that the lower ends of asparagus are tough and tasteless, so remove them by snapping them off prior to cooking. Bend the asparagus, and it will break at the exact point where the tender part ends and the fibrous part begins.

Ingredients

2 teaspoons olive oil

1 pound green asparagus, washed thoroughly, fibrous parts removed

1/4 teaspoon kosher salt

Freshly ground black pepper, to taste

2 teaspoons filtered water

Juice of 1/2 lemon

Cooking Instructions

1. Preheat the oil in a pan on medium high. (If preparing as a side dish to filet mignon, reheat the pan used for filet mignon.) When the oil begins to sizzle, carefully place the asparagus into the pan and sauté for 1 to 2 minutes on all sides. When asparagus is browned throughout, add the salt and pepper.
2. Add water and reduce the heat to low. Cover the pan and allow the asparagus to steam for 3 to 5 minutes, until the stalks soften but retain some of their crunch.
3. Turn off the heat and remove the lid. Sprinkle with lemon juice. Serve hot, at room temperature, or cold.

Prep and cooking time: 20 minutes
Serves 8

Cucumber and Bean Sprout Salad

This light summer salad is perfect for grilled fish. To dress it up even more, add any combination of cherry tomatoes, daikon radishes, shredded carrots, avocado, and basil, mint, or cilantro leaves.

Ingredients

1/2 cup arugula

1/2 English cucumber, scrubbed and thinly sliced

1/2 shallot, sliced

1/2 cup bean sprouts

1 tablespoon ponzu sauce

1 teaspoon sriracha

1 tablespoon avocado oil

Cooking Instructions

1. Combine arugula, cucumber, shallot, bean sprouts, and other herbs or vegetables you are using in a large bowl.
2. In a small bowl, whisk ponzu, sriracha, and avocado oil until the dressing is emulsified. Pour over the salad and mix thoroughly. Serve immediately.

Prep and cooking time: 10–12 minutes
Serves 2

Pacific Rim Slaw

This is a coleslaw with a twist—it uses delicate vegetables and dresses them with a substantive condiment inspired by Southeast Asian cuisines. The components of the dressing vary country to country, but they usually include some combination of the following: peanut butter, ginger, garlic, soy sauce, fish sauce, ponzu, vinegar, sesame oil, honey, scallions, and hot peppers. This mix presents a dizzying contrast in sour and sweet, salty and spicy. The Dubrow Diet is mostly free of sweeteners, but we are adding a teaspoon of honey here to balance the acidity of the lime juice and vinegar. You won't taste the sweetness, but you'll appreciate the goodness.

Ingredients

For the Slaw Mix:

1 small head napa cabbage, cored, washed, and shredded

1 small radicchio cabbage, thinly sliced

1 shallot, thinly sliced

2 sprigs of scallion, green and white parts, thinly sliced

1/2 cup julienned carrots

1 tablespoon sesame seeds

1 Hass avocado, pitted and cut into bite-size chunks

For the Dressing:

2 teaspoons almond butter

1 tablespoon low-sodium soy sauce

1 teaspoon honey (optional)

Juice of 1 lime

1 teaspoon sriracha

1/4 teaspoon kosher salt

1 tablespoon red wine vinegar

1 tablespoon olive oil

Cooking Instructions

1. In a salad bowl, combine the cabbages, shallot, scallion, and carrots.
2. In a medium-size bowl, whisk almond butter, soy sauce, honey, and lime juice until it reaches smooth and rich consistency. Add sriracha, salt, and vinegar and continue whisking. Add olive oil in a thin, steady stream until all the ingredients are fully integrated.
3. Pour the dressing into the salad and mix thoroughly. Top with sesame seeds and avocado chunks and serve immediately.

Prep time: 15–20 minutes
Serves 4 to 6

"Riced" Cauliflower

These days you can find riced cauliflower in the frozen section of your grocery store for twice the cost of a fresh head of cauliflower in the vegetable aisle. You'll never regret buying a head of cauliflower and ricing it yourself in a large food processor right before cooking. It will be fresher and less bitter to taste. Cauliflower comes in different sizes, and you can't trust your eyes to estimate how much you'll need. A medium-size head will yield 3 cups of riced florets, which will reduce to about half its original volume while cooking. On average, it will serve two to four people, more if you add other vegetables to it. If your cauliflower measurement is off, no worries: riced cauliflower isn't a science. Half a cup more or less won't make or break a dish. Besides, you can always adjust the seasoning.

Ingredients

Florets of 1 medium head of cauliflower, trimmed and washed

Canola oil spray

1/4 teaspoon kosher salt

Freshly ground black pepper, to taste

Cooking Instructions

1. Rice cauliflower florets in a large food processor, pulsing 3 or 4 times until the mixture reaches a grainy consistency. Between pulsing, use a plastic spatula to move the larger pieces closer to the blade so they too can be chopped. Don't overprocess; the mixture can become soupy.
2. Preheat a medium or large nonstick pan. Spray with canola oil. Place the cauliflower in the pan, slightly flattened to prevent over steaming. Add salt and pepper. Sauté until it starts toasting and softening, for 5 to 7 minutes. Don't overcook; you want the "rice" to be a touch crunchy. Serve immediately, at room temperature, or cold with left-over meat, chicken, or seafood.

Prep and cooking time: 12–15 minutes
Serves 4

"Riced" Cauliflower, Chinese Style

You'll never miss rice with this creative vegetable substitution. As easily adaptable to any cooking style or tradition as rice, riced cauliflower can be made Asian, Indian, or Mediterranean style by changing the spices and aromatic herbs. Keep in mind that the cauliflower volume decreases to half its original size when sautéed.

Ingredients

Florets of 1 medium head of cauliflower, trimmed and washed

2 tablespoons olive oil, divided

6–8 sweet mini bell peppers or 1 red bell pepper, stems and seeds removed and flesh cubed

3 to 4 bok choy clusters, trimmed, thoroughly washed, and sliced into strips

1-inch fresh ginger, peeled and chopped

2 cloves garlic, chopped

2 sprigs of green onion, green and white parts divided

1/2 teaspoon kosher salt

1/2 teaspoon Chinese five-spice powder

1 tablespoon tamari sauce

1 tablespoon toasted sesame seeds

Cooking Instructions

1. In a food processor, pulse cauliflower florets until they reach grain-like consistency. Don't over-pulse, as you don't want to turn these florets into baby food.
2. Preheat the pan and brush with half the oil. Stir-fry, for 2 to 3 minutes, the peppers, bok choy, fresh ginger, garlic, and the white parts of the scallions.
3. When the peppers are soft, add the cauliflower, salt, and five-spice powder. Fold in carefully and cook for another 3 minutes until the cauliflower softens and browns but retains some of its crunch.
4. Turn off the heat and add tamari sauce, stirring carefully.
5. Sprinkle with sesame seeds and serve as a side dish for Tri Tip Steak (p. 157), chicken, shrimp, fish, or meatballs. Refrigerate the leftovers and enjoy it cold, too.

Prep and cooking time: 20–25 minutes
Serves 4–6 as a side dish

Curried Cauliflower "Rice," Indian Style

In India, every family has its own signature curry spice, and the same goes for grocery stores here that carry varieties in degrees of spiciness and color, which range from pumpkin yellow to red and garnet. Whichever you choose will work for this recipe; just make sure you place it into the pan 1 teaspoon at a time and taste before adding more.

Ingredients

Florets of 1 medium head of cauliflower, trimmed and washed
2 tablespoons olive oil
2-inch fresh ginger, peeled and diced
3 cloves garlic, finely chopped
shallot, finely chopped
1/2 teaspoon kosher salt
2 teaspoons curry powder
1 tablespoon coconut cream
2 tablespoons fresh mint leaves, diced

Cooking Instructions

1. Pulse the cauliflower florets in a large food processor until the mixture reaches grainy consistency. Don't over-process or it will turn soupy.
2. Heat the oil in a nonstick pan on medium high. Add the ginger, garlic, shallot, and salt and sauté until the shallot begins to soften, about 2 to 3 minutes.
3. Add the cauliflower and sauté, stirring intermittently with a wooden or silicon spoon, for 5 to 7 minutes until the riced florets soften and crisp. They should retain some of the crunch and maybe even toast a little at the bottom for extra chewy texture. Stir in the curry and the coconut cream and allow to steam for 1 to 2 minutes. Garnish with mint and serve immediately, at room temperature, or cold.

Prep and cooking time: 15–20 minutes
Makes 1½ cups; serves 2–4 as a side dish

Cauliflower "Rice," Mediterranean Style

Mediterranean cuisine refers to a multitude of cultures ranging from Italy, Greece, and France to Morocco, Lebanon, and Israel. Here we are calling this riced cauliflower "Mediterranean" because it utilizes the staple regional ingredients of olives, lemon, and garlic. If you are looking for a different kind of Mediterranean, you can always play with spices and aromatic herbs like rosemary, cumin, sage, oregano, basil, or leeks. Cauliflower will absorb all flavors most graciously.

Ingredients

Florets of 1 medium head of cauliflower, trimmed and washed

2 tablespoons olive oil

3 cloves garlic, finely chopped

1 shallot, finely chopped

1/2 teaspoon kosher salt

1/2 teaspoon paprika

3 tablespoons capers, chopped

6 Sicilian olives, pitted and chopped

3 radicchio leaves, thinly sliced

2 tablespoons fresh parsley leaves, finely chopped

Juice of 1/2 lemon

Cooking Instructions

1. "Rice" the cauliflower by pulsing the florets in a large food processor until they reach grainy consistency. Don't over-pulse or the mixture will turn soupy.
2. Heat the olive oil in a nonstick pan on medium high. Add the garlic, shallot, and salt and sauté until the shallot softens, about 2 to 3 minutes.
3. Add the riced cauliflower to the pan and sauté, stirring intermittently, until the cauliflower softens and starts to toast, about 5 to 7 minutes. Add paprika, capers, and olives, mix thoroughly, and sauté for another minute longer; then turn off the heat.
4. Mix in strips of radicchio and parsley leaves, allowing them to wilt. Sprinkle with lemon juice right before serving. Serve immediately.

Prep and cooking time: 20–25 minutes
Serves 2–4 as a side dish

Main Meal Proteins

Petite Filet Mignon

If you are wondering what the difference is between a regular filet mignon and a petite one, the answer is in the question: in a petite filet mignon, the loin is smaller in diameter, between 2 and 4 inches when raw. Filet mignon is the most luxurious, tender, and expensive cut of meat, and when prepared correctly it will practically melt in your mouth. The good news is that if you are on an intermittent fasting diet, you don't have to have much to feel satiated. Beef tenderloin (from which filet mignon comes) is delicious enough naturally not to require a lot of dressing or spices to make it memorable, but if you have some fresh rosemary, thyme, and sage leaves, this is a great opportunity to use them. Serve the tenderloin with Pan-Seared Asparagus (p. 176) and a drizzle of Basic Chimichurri Sauce (p. 194) for a family meal or a special occasion.

Ingredients

1½ pounds petite filet mignon

1 tablespoon olive oil

1/4 teaspoon kosher salt

Freshly ground black pepper, to taste

3–5 sprigs of fresh rosemary, thyme, and bay leaves (optional)

Cooking Instructions

1. Preheat the oven to 375 degrees. Line a baking sheet with aluminum foil or parchment paper.
2. Unwrap the tenderloin (retain the twine) and pat dry with a paper towel to absorb excess moisture.
3. Brush the tenderloin with oil on all sides and sprinkle with salt and pepper.
4. On the stovetop, heat a nonstick pan large enough to hold the loin. Using tongs, transfer the loin to the pan and sear on medium high heat until the meat is browned all over, about 1 to 2 minutes per side.
5. Transfer the tenderloin to the lined baking sheet.

6. Place the fresh herbs, if using, underneath the twine holding the tenderloin. Bake for 12 minutes. Remove from the oven and allow to rest for 5 to 7 minutes.
7. Remove the twine with scissors and, using a sharp knife, slice the tenderloin into 2-inch rounds. The meat should be fairly rare. Return the filets to the baking sheet and bake for another 5 minutes for medium rare. Serve immediately.

Prep and cooking time: 35–40 minutes
Serves 8

Baked Salmon Fillets

A salmon fillet is a versatile staple of a healthy American diet and can be enjoyed with a simple seasoning of salt and pepper and consumed warm, at room temperature, or cold. It can be the main attraction as an entrée with a side dish or used as a salad topping. A superior source of protein and good fats, a salmon fillet can be cooked on a stovetop, in an oven, or on a grill (best done on a piece of aluminum foil or on a soaked cedar plank). There are countless ways to cook a salmon fillet, but this one is a reliable crowd-pleaser and weight-management aid. Keep an eye on it as it bakes; when the flesh begins to flake, it is safe to remove the salmon from the oven. Salmon tends to lose its silkiness when it is overcooked.

Ingredients

Olive or canola oil spray

6 fresh salmon fillets, 4 to 6 ounces each

1/2 teaspoon kosher salt

Freshly ground black pepper, to taste

1 tablespoon ground fennel seeds

1 tablespoon whole-grain mustard

1/4 cup fresh dill leaves

1/4 cup fresh parsley leaves

3 anchovy fillets (optional)

Juice of 1 lemon

2 tablespoons olive oil

Cooking Instructions

1. Preheat the oven to 400. Line a baking sheet with aluminum foil or parchment paper and spray with olive or canola oil to prevent sticking.
2. Place the salmon, skin-side down, on the lined baking sheet. Season with salt, pepper, and fennel seed.
3. In a small food processor, pulse the mustard, fresh herbs, anchovy fillets (if using), lemon juice, and oil. Brush the fillets with the mixture. Bake for 10 to 12 minutes for medium rare or 3 more minutes if you want your fillets well done.
4. Remove from the oven and allow to rest for 5 minutes before serving. Serve the salmon fillets with or without skin on, whatever your preference. It is easiest to keep the fillets intact by serving them with a wide stainless-steel spatula.

Prep and cooking time: 20 minutes
Serves 6

Sesame Seed Crusted Seared Tuna

This quick and easy to cook pan-seared tuna is crusted with a mix of black and white sesame seeds (called "tuxedo"), which make it a colorful centerpiece on a plate next to a cucumber and sprout salad or any green vegetables. Don't worry—you don't have to run out to buy a prepared mix of black and white sesame seeds. Any color of sesame seeds will do; they just look better in combination. For this recipe, splurge on sushi-quality tuna, as it is seared on both sides but remains rare on the inside. If raw tuna isn't your cup of tea, so to speak, then you may just as well eat it out of a can (but only if it is packed in water). We use Spike, one of our favorite salt-free seasonings, with this recipe. You won't miss the salt, especially if you serve the tuna with our Cucumber and Bean Sprout Salad (p. 176), which is saltier.

Ingredients

2 fresh tuna fillets, 6 ounces each

1/2 teaspoon Spike seasoning

1 tablespoon olive oil, divided

1/4 cup black and white sesame seeds

Cooking Instructions

1. Dab the tuna fillets with a paper towel to absorb excess moisture. Season on both sides with Spike.
2. Preheat half the olive oil on high heat in a nonstick pan until it sizzles. (Fish fillets crisp up faster on high heat.)
3. While the oil is heating up, scatter the sesame seeds on a large plate. Dip the tuna fillets into the seeds on both sides. They should stick, making a nice, thick crust. Discard any excess sesame seeds.
4. Carefully place the fillets into the pan to avoid oil splattering (but keep your distance just in case). Lower the heat to medium high and sear for 1 to 2 minutes per side. Slice the tuna into 1/2-inch strips and serve immediately.

Prep and cooking time: 10–12 minutes
Serves 2

Classic Meatballs

These classic meatballs are delicious on their own or dressed with either our Classic Marinara Sauce (p. 195) or Quick Romesco Sauce (p. 196). They also make a great companion for riced cauliflower or spaghetti squash. Freeze the leftovers, if any, for up to a month. For this recipe, you can also use ground bison meat. Keep in mind that meatballs are cooked in batches, and the number of batches will depend on the size of the sauté pan you are using. If you are using a standard three-quart pan, you should cook the meatballs in this recipe in three batches for optimal results. But don't get hung up on the size of the pan; just make sure that you don't overcrowd the meatballs when you sear them, and add enough oil to each batch to avoid sticking and burning.

Ingredients

1/2 red onion, roughly chopped

1/2 cup fresh parsley leaves

1 teaspoon plus 3 tablespoons olive oil, divided; more if needed

1 pound ground beef

1/2 teaspoon salt

1/4 teaspoon freshly ground black pepper

1 egg

Cooking Instructions

1. In a small food processor, blend onion and parsley leaves with 1 teaspoon of the olive oil until liquefied.
2. In a medium bowl, place the ground beef, onion/parsley blend, salt and pepper, and egg. Mix thoroughly—but don't overmix—using your hands (wash them thoroughly before and after) or a silicone spatula until the mixture is uniform. Cover and refrigerate for 1/2 hour.
3. Remove the meat mixture from the refrigerator. Make 1½-inch meatballs by rolling the meat into smooth spheres by hand. Keep a bowl of cold water nearby to dip your hands in to make them less sticky. Lay out the meatballs on a plastic cutting board or a large plate.
4. Preheat 1 tablespoon of oil in a nonstick pan. When the oil begins to sizzle, place the meatballs in the pan, taking care not to be burned by splattering oil. Don't overcrowd the meatballs. It is best to sear them in batches, with one tablespoon of oil at a time. Depending on the size of the pan you are using, you should have 2 to 3 batches.
5. The meatballs need to brown on each side, which can take anywhere from 30 seconds to a minute depending on your pan and heat levels. Don't step away from the pan while the meatballs are browning. Turn the meatballs over by jiggling the handle of the pan in a way that makes them flip. You don't have to be Julia Child to accomplish this maneuver, but it does require some experience. You can also flip them using a flat or slotted stainless-steel spatula. Don't press down on the meatballs or you will release all the juices. Try not to keep the meatballs cooking for more than 3 minutes per batch or they may overcook.
6. Using a slotted spoon or spatula, carefully place the meatballs into a clean container until all the batches are done. Then move the entire batch back into the pan. Turn off the heat and keep the pan covered for 3 to 5 minutes, allowing the inside of the meatballs to cook through by

steaming in their own juices. Serve hot on top of "Riced" Cauliflower (p. 178) or "zoodles" of spaghetti squash, or reheated with Classic Marinara Sauce (p. 195) or Quick Romesco Sauce (p. 196).

Prep and cooking time: 1 hour, more for cooling in the refrigerator
Serves 6

Squashes, Soups, and a Chili, Too

Pad Thai Zoodles

Pad thai is a dish voluptuous in flavor and impact; eat it too often and watch your waistline expand. This dish is a creative variation that preserves the tastes of saltiness, sweetness, sourness, and spice, but without the guilt. Instead of noodles, we use spiralized zucchini, known as "zoodles." If you don't own a spiralizer, store-bought zoodles will do; just make sure you consume them shortly after buying because spiralized zucchini doesn't retain its freshness for long. You can buy sambal oelek chili paste, a classic Indonesian condiment, in the Asian section of most gourmet grocery stores, or order it on Amazon.com. You can substitute sriracha sauce for the sambal oelek. Sriracha tends to be spicier, so use it more sparingly. Instead of sugar, we use mirin, a Japanese rice wine, to cut down on the acidity of the ponzu.

Ingredients

1 tablespoon olive oil

3–5 zucchini, spiraled (zoodles)

1/2 teaspoon kosher salt

1 tablespoon sambal oelek paste

2 teaspoons mirin

1 tablespoon ponzu

1 tablespoon sesame oil

1 cup bean sprouts

1 sprig of scallion, diced, white and green parts separated

5 basil leaves, shredded (optional)

Cooking Instructions

1. Line a large plate with paper towels.
2. Heat the olive oil in a nonstick pan. Stir-fry the zoodles until they soften, 3 to 5 minutes. Place on the paper towel and sprinkle with salt. Allow the salt and the oil to drain from the zoodles as they cool to room temperature.
3. Make the dressing by whisking sambal oelek, mirin, ponzu, sesame oil, and white parts of the scallion.
4. Divide the zoodles and bean sprouts between two bowls. Pour half the dressing over each bowl and mix lightly.
5. Sprinkle with green parts of the scallions and the shredded basil, if using. Serve immediately.

Prep and cooking time: 12–15 minutes
Serves 2

Roasted Spaghetti Squash (Phase 2 only)

Spaghetti squash is stringy when cooked and resembles strands of ordinary spaghetti on the plate. Some people complain that spaghetti squash can be a little bland, but being naturally spongy, it sops up the juices of any food you place on top of it, which make it an ideal base for traditional tomato-based sauces like marinara or with meatballs. Be careful when slicing the raw squash, which is very hard. You'll need a sharp knife and a steady hand to do it right, or just have your grocer split the squash in half for you.

Ingredients

1 medium spaghetti squash, cut lengthwise

2 tablespoons olive oil

1 teaspoon kosher salt

Freshly ground black pepper, to taste

Cooking Instructions

1. Preheat the oven to 400 degrees. Line a baking sheet with aluminum foil or parchment paper.

2. Brush the inside of the squash with oil, then sprinkle with salt and pepper. Place on the lined baking sheet flesh-side down and roast for 50 to 60 minutes until the squash softens and releases some of its juices. Remove from the oven and cool completely.
3. After the squash is cool enough to handle, turn it over and scoop out and discard the seeds. Scoop out the flesh of the squash into a bowl. If it seems watery, drain the squash through a fine-meshed sieve.
4. Place the squash on serving plates. Slightly hollow out the middle. Serve with meatballs and marinara sauce.

Prep and cooking time: 1 hour 15 minutes, more to cool
Serves 4

A Tasty Touch of Thai Soup

What this soup lacks in creaminess it makes up for in its complex flavors and speed of preparation. If you don't have the time to make your own chicken broth from scratch, use a store-bought organic variety. Just keep in mind that not all commercial broths are alike, so you may have to adjust the amount of salt you use. There is no additional salt in this recipe because the fish sauce is quite salty, but it may not be enough if you are using a store-bought broth.

Ingredients

1 teaspoon sesame oil

1 serrano chili, sliced

2-inch fresh ginger, peeled

1 sprig of scallion, sliced, green and white parts separated

6 button mushrooms,

1 Roma tomato, diced, pulp removed

4 cups homemade or organic store-bought chicken broth

1 tablespoon fish sauce

1 cup baby kale

Juice of 1/2 lime

1 cup bean sprouts

12 shrimp, shell and tail off, cooked (optional)

5 fresh basil leaves, shredded

Cooking Instructions

1. Brush a preheated pot with sesame oil. Flash-sauté chili, ginger, white scallion parts, mushrooms, and tomato for 1 to 2 minutes.
2. Add the chicken broth and fish sauce and bring to a boil. Add kale and simmer, on low, until the greens wilt. Drizzle with lime juice.
3. Prepare four serving bowls. Divide the bean sprouts and shrimp (if using) evenly between them. Ladle the soup on top. Garnish with basil and serve immediately.

Prep and cooking time: 12–15 minutes
Serves 4 as a main dish, 6 as an appetizer

Jazzy Gazpacho

Over the centuries, this signature cold soup has been transported from its native Spain to that nation's former colonies around the world, including the Americas. During this journey, the gazpacho has been transformed in an infinite number of ways. Traditional recipes call for all the vegetables to be hand chopped to soupy consistency, a skill that requires a very sharp knife and a lot of time and experience. We are going to shortcut this process without coming up short on the divine layers of flavors.

Ingredients

2 tablespoons olive oil

1/2 red onion, sliced

1 red bell pepper, seeded and sliced

1 jalapeño pepper, stemmed, seeded, and roughly chopped

3 garlic cloves

Leaves from 3 sprigs of fresh tarragon

1 teaspoon kosher salt

1/2 teaspoon freshly ground black pepper

Sacramento or another variety of tomato juice, 46-ounce can or bottle

2 tablespoons red wine vinegar

5 Persian or Kirby cucumbers or 1 English seedless cucumber, finely diced

6 Roma or other medium-size tomatoes, cored and diced

Leaves from 3 sprigs of fresh mint, finely chopped

Cooking Instructions

1. Heat the oil in a nonstick sauté pan. When the oil begins to sizzle, add onion, bell and jalapeño peppers, garlic, tarragon, and salt and pepper and sauté until the vegetables soften, about 5 to 7 minutes. Allow to cool to room temperature.
2. Place the vegetables with a splash of tomato juice in a food processor or blender and puree until smooth.
3. Pour the mixture into a smooth bowl and whisk in the remainder of the tomato soup in batches until fully incorporated. Add the vinegar and whisk some more. Adjust seasoning.
4. Cover and refrigerate for at least 4 hours.
5. Mix the diced cucumbers, tomatoes, and mint leaves to create a kind of relish and refrigerate until you are ready to serve.
6. To serve, stir the cucumber tomato relish into the tomato juice/vegetable puree. You should see a chunky, bright soup. Adjust the seasoning one more time if needed and dive in.

Prep and cooking time: 45 minutes, more for cooling
Serves 10–12

Black Bean Chili

You can make this chili with ingredients already in your pantry, either as a standalone meal or part of a cookout. We use canned black beans here to speed up the process, but I recommend you use the organic variety to reduce the number of preservatives. Rinsing the beans will cleanse them even further. If you are in a rush, you can easily take an hour out of the process by sautéing the vegetables for less time and reducing the amount of time the beans bake in the oven, but the flavors will not be as deep. If you want to rev up the protein intake, add either ground turkey or ground beef at the end of the cooking process. Just sauté the meat for 3 minutes in a pan with a drizzle of olive oil, breaking it apart with a wooden spatula, and carefully move it into the pot of chili along with the other ingredients in step 3 of the cooking instructions.

Ingredients

2 tablespoons olive oil

1 large or 2 medium yellow onions, diced

1 green bell pepper

1 quart vegetable broth

Organic black beans, two 15-ounce cans, drained and rinsed thoroughly

1 teaspoon kosher salt

1/2 teaspoon freshly ground black pepper

1 teaspoon garlic powder

1/2 teaspoon ground cumin

1 teaspoon smoked paprika

1 teaspoon Mexican oregano

1 teaspoon ancho chili powder

1 chipotle chili pepper in adobe sauce, diced

3 San Marzano or other whole peeled tomatoes from a can, chopped

2 dry bay leaves

Cooking Instructions

1. Preheat the oven to 275 degrees.
2. Heat the olive oil in a thick-bottomed ovenproof pot, preferably a Dutch oven. When the oil begins to sizzle, add the onions and peppers. Cook on high heat for 5 to 7 minutes until the vegetables soften. Reduce the temperature to medium low and continue cooking, stirring frequently, for about 20 minutes. The longer you cook the vegetables, the more flavorful your chili will be. If they start sticking to the pan, drizzle them—repeatedly if needed—with vegetable broth.

3. Add the beans, spices, tomatoes, remaining vegetable broth, and bay leaves and bring to a boil on high heat. Skim the surface with a slotted spoon. Cover the pot and place in the oven. Bake for another 45 minutes to an hour, stirring occasionally to prevent sticking, until the chili reaches your desired consistency. Remember, the longer you cook it, the silkier and smokier it will become.
4. Remove from the oven and adjust seasoning. Discard the bay leaves. Serve immediately. Freeze the leftovers, if any.

Prep and cooking time: 2 hours
Serves 8–10

Sauces

Basic Chimichurri Sauce

This is a classic grilled meat condiment served in Argentina. The herb-infused sauce nicely balances red meat cooked on a grill or stovetop.

Ingredients

1 cup fresh parsley leaves, washed thoroughly and loosely packed

1 garlic clove

1 jalapeño pepper, stemmed and seeded

1/2 teaspoon kosher salt

2 teaspoons red wine vinegar

1 tablespoon olive oil

Cooking Instructions

1. In a food processor, pulse the parsley leaves, garlic, jalapeño pepper, salt, and vinegar. When the mixture becomes grainy, pulse again while pouring oil into the processor in a thin stream.
2. Place into a covered bowl and refrigerate until you are ready to use. Drizzle over meat or vegetables, a teaspoon or two per serving.

Prep and cooking time: 5–10 minutes
Makes 1/3 cup

Classic Marinara Sauce

Marinara sauce is easy to find at a grocery store in commercially produced varieties as well as more gourmet options. We don't mind if you use a store-bought marinara for your spaghetti squash or meatballs, but remember that they contain a lot of sugar to counterbalance the natural acidity of tomatoes. We sweeten our tomatoes with carrots and no other sugary additives. So, if you have some time on your hands, this sauce is easy to make and freezes nicely for later use.

Ingredients

2 tablespoons olive oil

1 large or 2 medium yellow onions, finely diced

2 celery sticks, finely diced

2 carrots, peeled and finely grated

5 garlic cloves, finely diced

1 teaspoon kosher salt

1/4 teaspoon freshly ground black pepper

1/2 teaspoon red chili flakes

1/2 teaspoon dried oregano

1/2 teaspoon dried basil

1 tablespoon tomato paste

8-ounce can tomato sauce

28-ounce can San Marzano or other peeled tomatoes

2 dry bay leaves

Cooking Instructions

1. Heat the oil in a large thick-bottomed pan, preferably a Dutch oven. When the oil begins to sizzle, add the onions, celery, carrots, garlic cloves, and salt and sauté on medium high heat until the vegetables have softened and browned, about 15 to 20 minutes, stirring frequently to prevent burning. Splash with water if they start sticking.
2. Add the pepper, chili flakes, oregano, and basil and mix thoroughly. Add the tomato paste, tomato sauce, and tomatoes from the can, one

ingredient at a time, mixing the sauce thoroughly in between. Continue simmering for 10 minutes, slowly adding drizzles of sauce from the can of tomatoes to add moisture.

3. Add the bay leaves and continue simmering on low heat, uncovered, for 30 minutes to 1½ hours, if you have time. The longer it cooks, the more delicious it will be. If you feel the moisture is evaporating too quickly, just add more water to it, 1/3 cup at a time. Adjust seasonings and serve hot.

Prep and cooking time: 1 hour 30 minutes, more if you simmer longer
Serves 12

Quick Romesco Sauce

This sauce is naturally smoky because the tomatoes and peppers are grilled or broiled, but in this recipe we shortcut the process with store-bought peppers and tomato sauce. We've added smokiness with paprika and replaced the bread crumbs with the healthier sunflower seeds. Use it as cocktail sauce for shrimp, to dress up meatballs, or as a dollop of flavor on grilled meats or sturdy steamed veggies like broccoli, cabbage, string beans, or asparagus.

Ingredients

1/3 cup toasted sunflower seeds
2 tablespoons fresh parsley leaves
2 jarred red bell peppers, rinsed
1 jarred pimento pepper, rinsed
2 tablespoons tomato sauce
1 tablespoon sherry vinegar
1/4 teaspoon kosher salt
1 teaspoon Hungarian smoked paprika
1/4 teaspoon ground coriander
2 tablespoons olive oil

Cooking Instructions

1. Toast the sunflower seeds on medium high heat in a nonstick pan for about 3 to 4 minutes, until they start browning. Place into a clean bowl to stop the toasting. Seeds burn quickly.
2. Place the sunflower seeds in a food processor and pulse until it reaches a pasty consistency, on the edge of buttery. Add the parsley leaves and pulse until integrated.
3. Add peppers, tomato sauce, vinegar, salt, and spices and pulse while pouring the olive oil in a stream until the mixture becomes saucy. Adjust spices if needed. Refrigerate for at least an hour prior to serving.

Prep and cooking time: 10–15 minutes, more for cooling.
Makes 1½ cups

Smoothies and Desserts

A Virgin Piña Colada with Benefits Smoothie (Phase 2 Only)

This green smoothie has a hint of exotic, fruity smoothness that is filling enough to be a full meal, especially after fasting.

Ingredients

1 cup baby spinach

1 cup filtered water

1 cup mango

5-ounce container plain coconut yogurt

Instructions

Place the ingredients in a blender and puree until the smoothie is silky green.

Prep time: 5–10 minutes
Serves 2–4

A Savory Smoothie

This smoothie comes with a topping of lemon zest, grated cucumber, freshly ground black pepper, and sumac, in case you want to serve it for a more formal breakfast or brunch. Sumac is a Middle Eastern spice that adds smokiness and sourness to vegetables and gives any dish a beautiful garnet-colored sprinkle. If you are not into sour, then reduce the amount of lemon zest. Cashewgurt is a dairy-free yogurt made with cashews.

Ingredients

Zest and juice of 1 lemon

1/2 avocado

2/3 English cucumber, divided in half, sliced and grated

Fresh mint leaves from 2 sprigs

1/4 teaspoon kosher salt, divided

1 cup cashewgurt*

1 cup baby kale

1 cup filtered water

Freshly ground black pepper, to taste

1/8 teaspoon sumac

Instructions

1. Place lemon juice, avocado, cucumber slices, mint leaves, half the salt, cashewgurt, kale, and water into a blender and puree until smooth.
2. Divide into serving glasses. Top with pepper, the remaining salt, lemon zest, sumac, and grated cucumber. Serve immediately.

Prep time: 10–15 minutes
Serves 4

Morning Glory (lime papaya smoothie or ice pops)

Papaya is a great fruit for weight loss because it is relatively low in sugar, and while it is watery, it is always filling. Lime enhances its earthy

---

*If you can't find cashewgurt, try plain kefir as an alternative. Note that plain kefir is a little on the sour side.

freshness, and ginger gives it a bit of a bite. You can enjoy this recipe as a smoothie or dessert in a form of an ice pop. If you've never bought a fresh papaya, select one as you would a ripe avocado—not too soft (you don't want it to be spotty or have indentation marks), but not too hard.

Ingredients

1 medium papaya, ripe, peeled, seeded, and roughly chopped

Juice of 1 lime

1 Bartlett pear, stem and seeds removed, roughly chopped

1 kiwi, peeled

1-inch fresh ginger, peeled

3 fresh basil leaves

1/4 cup filtered water

1 cup ice (if making smoothies, not ice pops)

Instructions

Place all the ingredients except the ice in a blender and puree until smooth. If you are making ice pops, pour into a mold and freeze for at least 4 hours before serving. If you are making a smoothie, place the ice into the blender and crush until the smoothie reaches your desired consistency. Pour into glasses and serve immediately.

Prep time: 7–10 minutes
Serves 4 (smoothies) or 8 (ice pops)

Banana Grape Chia Pudding (smoothie or dessert) (Phase 3 only)

This dairy-free fruit smoothie is sweetened with all-natural ingredients and thickened with nutrient-dense chia seeds, which give the smoothie a creamy texture of pudding. Cashewgurt—a dairy-free yogurt derived from cashews—makes this indulgence a vegan alternative to the more conventional dairy smoothie options.

Ingredients

1 banana

6 ounces seedless grapes

1 cup cashewgurt*

2 tablespoons chia seeds

Instructions

1. In a blender, puree banana and grapes until they reach a juicy consistency.
2. Add cashewgurt and pulse until well blended.
3. Divide between two serving bowls, cups, or glasses. Add a teaspoon of chia seeds into each serving and stir thoroughly. Leave for 15 minutes to gel. Serve immediately or refrigerate up to 2 hours.

Prep time: 5 minutes, more for waiting time
Serves 2

Peaches and "Cream"

This easy to prepare summer dessert is completely sugar, grain, dairy, and gluten free. It is served in fresh peach halves that can either be grilled or baked. The filling is coconut based, but keep in mind that coconut products have natural and healthy fats so it should be consumed sparingly. (We recommend 1 to 2 tablespoons per serving.) The spice mix gives it an exotic and refreshing flavor. The dessert will take minutes to make but requires an overnight straining of the yogurt, so think of this as a planned-in-advance indulgence to be savored. How much "cream" is yielded from the yogurt will depend upon the thickness of the yogurt used; a thicker variety is best.

Ingredients

8 ounces coconut yogurt (yields 1/3 to 1 cup cream, depending upon yogurt thickness)

Zest of 1 lemon

1/4 teaspoon vanilla

1/4 teaspoon ground cinnamon

1/4 teaspoon ground cardamom

---

*If you can't find cashewgurt, try plain kefir as an alternative. Note that plain kefir is a little on the sour side.

2 peaches, halved and pitted immediately prior to grilling

Grapeseed oil spray

1 tablespoon crushed pecans

Fresh mint leaves for garnish

Instructions

1. Stack a metal strainer over a glass bowl. Line the strainer with cheesecloth and carefully pour in the coconut yogurt. Tie the cloth and, leaving it over the bowl, place in the refrigerator to strain overnight.
2. Once the yogurt has been strained (the cream should be a third of the yogurt's original volume), place it in a dish and whisk in the lemon zest, vanilla, cinnamon, and cardamom. Cover with plastic wrap and return to refrigerator.
3. To grill the peaches, heat a nonstick grill brushed with grapeseed oil. Grill the peaches 4 minutes on each side. Remove from the grill and allow to cool completely.
4. To serve, top each peach half with 1 to 2 tablespoons of coconut cream topping and sprinkle with crushed pecans. Top with fresh mint leaves if desired for optimal presentation.

Prep time: 15 minutes, plus overnight yogurt straining
Serves 4

A Berry Tartlet (Phase 2 only)

A simple dessert can be full of guilt-free natural goodness. We've kept the processed sugar out of this treat, but if berries make a filling that's too tart for your taste, then add a tablespoon of anti-inflammatory manuka honey. It will not make it too sweet, but it will temper the acidity. The tart shell is made with almond and rye flour, coconut oil, and eggs. If you are gluten intolerant, note that rye flour is not gluten-free, but it is lower in gluten than wheat flour, and it has the benefits of anti-inflammatory properties. The tartlets can be made in a regular 12-piece muffin baking dish. Because it is mostly gluten-free, the shell can be challenging to roll out, but you can patch it together using your fingers. It doesn't have to be perfect, as it will come out of the muffin tin intact after baking. The filling can be prepared up to a day in advance. For a more formal presentation, serve the Berry Tartlets with a coconut whip cream on top.

For the Tart Shell:

Ingredients

1 cup barley flour

1 cup almond flour

1/4 teaspoon kosher salt

1/2 cup coconut oil

2 large eggs

Canola spray oil (for the pan)

Cooking Instructions

Prepare the batter by sifting the flours and salt into a large bowl. Using a pastry cutter, integrate the coconut oil into the flour until the mixture becomes pebbly. Whisk in the eggs until the batter turns sticky and clay-like. Form the batter into a log, wrap in plastic, and refrigerate until ready to use, but at least for 1/2 hour.

For the Filling:

Ingredients

20 ounces frozen berries

1 cup filtered water

4 ounces seedless grapes

1 tablespoon manuka honey (optional)

1 tablespoon almond flour

Cooking Instructions

1. In a heavy-bottomed pan or Dutch oven, bring the berries, water, grapes, and honey, if using, to a boil. Reduce heat to medium low and simmer, covered, for 15 to 20 minutes until the mixture thickens and most of the water evaporates.
2. Add flour, stir to combine, and simmer for another 3 minutes. Remove from heat and allow to cool to room temperature.

Baking Instructions

1. Preheat the oven to 400 degrees. Dust a large, preferably wooden cutting board with a tablespoon of flour. Spray a muffin pan with canola oil.
2. Remove the dough from the wrap and slice into 12 even pieces. Using a rolling pin, also lightly dusted in flour, do your best to roll out the shells one at a time.
3. Carefully deposit the raw tart shells into the cups of the muffin pan, pressing down with your fingers to make sure it fits snuggly around the tin. Be patient with the dough, as it will try to break apart. If it does, patch it inside the muffin cups with your hands.
4. Bake the shells for 15 minutes. Remove from the oven. Lower the temperature to 350 degrees.
5. Using a spoon, distribute the filling among the tart shells, filling each one 2/3 of the way up. Bake for another 12 minutes and remove from the oven. Cool completely before serving. Serve as is or with a dollop of coconut whip cream.

Prep and cooking time: 1½ hours
Serves 12

"Naked" Baked Apples

My sorority sisters and I used to make a version of this delicious dessert in college, and even though none of us could really cook, it seemed to always satisfy our craving for sweetness. Since we are not adding sugar to desserts, it is best to use a naturally sweet, sturdy apple variety such as Rome, Crispin, or Jonathans. The apple juices will caramelize while baking and the spices will give it richness without any additional calories. A glass casserole is optimal for capturing and retaining the apple juices for basting.

Ingredients

4 firm, sweet apples (Rome, Crispin, Jonathan)

1/4 teaspoon cinnamon

1/8 teaspoon ground cloves

1 star anise

3/4 cup white wine

Cooking Instructions

1. Preheat the oven to 375 degrees. Cut about an inch off each apple top and scoop out the seeds with the tip of a paring knife. Retain the tops.
2. Place the apples, bottom-side down, in a 9 × 9-inch casserole dish. Sprinkle the spices into the cavity of each apple and close each one with a top. Place the star anise in the middle of the dish and pour the wine around the apples. Bake for 45 to 55 minutes, basting the apples occasionally with the wine and juices at the bottom of the pan.
3. Remove from the oven and baste the apples with the baking juice, if any remains. Bring to room temperature before serving.

Prep and cooking time: 1 hour
Serves 4

Apples and Spice and Everything Nice

It's impossible not to love this original baked apple dish in which apples are stuffed with a jammy reduction of more apples, plums, spices, and oatmeal. The sourness of Granny Smith apples gives this dessert a distinctly grown-up designation, but if you do want it on the sweeter side, stick to more sugary apple variety such as Gala or Golden Delicious for the stuffing and add banana juice* to the mixture (see note). If you can't find Italian plums, any large, sturdy, sweet plum will do. In place of steel-cut oats, feel free to substitute quick-cooking oats, but not instant oatmeal. You can make the stuffing in advance, and if you have any leftovers, enjoy it as a snack the next day.

---

*To make banana water, place two peeled bananas in a glass bowl and microwave for 4 minutes, 2 minutes at a time. Be careful handling hot bananas. Line a clean bowl with a fine-meshed strainer. Place the bananas and their juice in the strainer and allow to drain for 15 minutes. Use the banana juice as sweetener in the stuffing. Don't discard the bananas; instead, cool them completely and mash into Greek yogurt or oatmeal for the non-dieters in your family. If you top the banana-laced yogurt or oatmeal with pecans and coconut flakes, it will be a breakfast or snack to remember. Serve immediately.

Ingredients

8 Apples: 4 for stuffing (any combination) and 4 for baking (preferably Granny Smith)

4 Italian plums, pitted and roughly chopped

1/4 teaspoon baking spice

2 ripe bananas (optional)*

1 tablespoon steel-cut oats

1 cup water

3/4 cup white wine

4 cinnamon sticks (optional)

Cooking Instructions

1. Peel, core, and chop the four apples for stuffing.
2. In a thick-bottomed pot or sauce pan, combine apples, plums, baking spice, banana juice (if using), oats, and water and bring to a boil. Reduce heat and simmer, covered, for 1 hour, stirring periodically with a wooden spoon to prevent sticking. The mixture should thicken and reduce to 1/3 its original volume, but it can still be a touch runny. Remove from heat and allow to cool to room temperature before moving to the next step. Refrigerate if you want to finish the dish later.
3. Preheat the oven to 375 degrees. Cut approximately 2 inches off the top of the 4 baking apples. Scoop out the seeds with a paring knife and hollow out the interior to make extra room for the stuffing. Slice some of the skin and flesh off the bottom of the baking apples, just enough to flatten them so they don't tip over in the baking pan.
4. Line up the baking apples in a glass 9 × 9-inch casserole. Using a tablespoon, place the stuffing into the cavity of each apple, just enough to fill it to the rim. If you have any left over, you won't be able to resist gobbling it up.
5. Ladle the wine on the bottom of the pan and bake, uncovered, for 45 minutes to an hour until the topping starts crusting over and the

baking apples begin to shrivel. Remove from the oven and place a cinnamon stick into the stuffing of each apple to give it that dapper look. Serve at room temperature.

Prep and cooking time: 2 hours, divided
Serves 4

Selected References

Introduction

Nobelprize.org, "The 2016 Nobel Prize in Physiology or Medicine," press release, October 3, 2016, http://www.nobelprize.org/nobel_prizes/medicine/laureates/2016/press.html.

Heilbronn, L. K., et. al. "Alternate-Day Fasting in Nonobese Subjects: Effects on Body Weight, Body Composition, and Energy Metabolism." *American Journal of Clinical Nutrition* 81, no. 1 (2005): 69–73.

Youm, Y. H., et al. "The Ketone Metabolite β-Hydroxybutyrate Blocks NLRP3 Inflammasome–Mediated Inflammatory Disease" *Nature Medicine* 21, no. 3 (2015): 263–269. doi:10.1038/nm.3804.

Mattson, M. P., et al. "Impact of Intermittent Fasting on Health and Disease Processes." *Ageing Research Reviews* 39 (2017): 46–58. doi: 10.1016/j.arr.2016.10.005.

Chapter 1

Klempel, M. C. et al. "Intermittent Fasting Combined with Calorie Restriction Is Effective for Weight Loss and Cardio-Protection in Obese Women." *Nutrition Journal* 11 (2012): 98. doi: 10.1186/1475-2891-11-98.

Johnstone, A. M. "Fasting—The Ultimate Diet?" *Obesity Reviews* 8, no. 3 (2007): 211–222. doi:10.1111/j.1467-789X.2006.00266.x.

Varady, K. A., et al. "Short-Term Modified Alternate-Day Fasting: A Novel Dietary Strategy for Weight Loss and Cardioprotection in Obese Adults." *American Journal of Clinical Nutrition* 90, no. 5 (2009):

1138–1143; first published online September 30, 2009. doi:10.3945/ajcn.2009.28380.

Varady, K. A., et al. "Alternate Day Fasting for Weight Loss in Normal Weight and Overweight Subjects: A Randomized Controlled Trial." *Nutrition Journal* 12, no. 1 (2013): 146. doi: 10.1186/1475-2891-12-146.

Ho, K. Y., et al. "Fasting Enhances Growth Hormone Secretion and Amplifies the Complex Rhythms of Growth Hormone Secretion in Man." *Journal of Clinical Investigation* 81, no. 4 (1988): 968–975.

Hartman, M. L., et al. "Augmented Growth Hormone (GH) Secretory Burst Frequency and Amplitude Mediate Enhanced GH Secretion During a Two-Day Fast in Normal Men." *Journal of Clinical Endocrinology & Metabolism* 74, no. 4 (1992): 757–765. https://doi.org/10.1210/jcem.74.4.1548337

Barnosky, A. R., et al. "Intermittent Fasting vs. Daily Calorie Restriction for Type 2 Diabetes Prevention: A Review of Human Findings." *Translational Research* 164, no. 4 (2014): 302–311. doi: 10.1016/j.trsl.2014.05.013.

Mattson, M. P., et al. "Impact of Intermittent Fasting on Health and Disease Processes." *Ageing Research Reviews* 39 (2017): 46–58. doi: 10.1016/j.arr.2016.10.005.

Gustafsson, A. B., and R. M. Mentzer. "Autophagy: An Endogenous Survival Mechanism and Cardioprotective Response to Ischemic Stress." In *Autophagy in Health and Disease*, edited by Roberta A. Gottlieb, chapter 9. London: Academic Press, 2013.

Mattson, M. P. "Energy Intake, Meal Frequency, and Health: A Neurobiological Perspective."

Annual Review of Nutrition 25, no. 1 (2005): 237–260. doi: 10.1146/annurev.nutr.25.050304.092526.

Weir, H. J., et al. "Dietary Restriction and AMPK Increase Lifespan via Mitochondrial Network and Peroxisome Remodeling" *Cell Metabolism* 26, no. 6 (2017): 884–896.e5. doi: http://dx.doi.org/10.1016/j.cmet.2017.09.024.

Chapter 2

Hardy, K., et al. "The Importance of Dietary Carbohydrate in Human Evolution." *Quarterly Review of Biology* 90, no. 3 (2015): 251–268. https://doi.org/10.1086/682587.

Levitsky, D. A., and C. R. Pacanowski, "Effect of Skipping Breakfast on Subsequent Energy Intake." *Physiology & Behavior* 119 (2013): 9–16. doi: 10.1016/j.physbeh.2013.05.006.

Gaur, A., et al. "Role of Ventromedial Hypothalamus in High Fat Diet Induced Obesity in Male Rats: Association with Lipid Profile, Thyroid Profile, and Insulin Resistance." *Annals of Neurosciences* 21, no. 3 (2014): 104–107. doi: 10.5214/ans.0972.7531.210306.

Chapter 3

Nobelprize.org, "The 2016 Nobel Prize in Physiology or Medicine," press release, October 3, 2016, http://www.nobelprize.org/nobel_prizes/medicine/laureates/2016/press.html.

Khusial, R., et al. "A Role For Autophagy In Skin Aging." Presented at the Summer Meeting of the American Academy of Dermatology, New York City, August 2015.

Altshuler-Keylin, S., and S. Kajimura. "Mitochondrial Homeostasis in Adipose Tissue Remodeling Science Signaling." *Science Signaling* 10, no. 468 (2017). doi: 10.1126/scisignal.aai9248.

Lee, J., et al. "Autophagy, Mitochondria and Oxidative Stress: Cross-Talk and Redox Signalling." *Biochemical Journal* 441, no. 2 (2012): 523–540. doi: 10.1042/BJ20111451.

Chapter 4

Stenblom, E. L., et al. "Consumption of Thylakoid-Rich Spinach Extract Reduces Hunger, Increases Satiety and Reduces Cravings for Palatable Food In Overweight Women." *Appetite* 91, no. 1 (2015): 209–219. https://doi.org/10.1016/j.appet.2015.04.051.

Montelius, C., et al. "Body Weight Loss, Reduced Urge for Palatable Food and Increased Release of GLP-1 Through Daily Supplementation with Green-Plant Membranes for Three Months in Overweight

Women." *Appetite* 81, no. 1: 295–304. https://doi.org/10.1016/j.appet.2014.06.101.

Benoit, S. C., et al. "Palmitic Acid Mediates Hypothalamic Insulin Resistance by Altering PKC-Θ Subcellular Localization in Rodents." *Journal of Clinical Investigation* 119, no. 9 (2009): 2577–2589. doi:10.1172/JCI36714.

Chapter 6

Bell, S. "Association Between Clinically Recorded Alcohol Consumption and Initial Presentation of 12 Cardiovascular Diseases: Population Based Cohort Study Using Linked Health Records." *BMJ* 356 (2017). doi: https://doi.org/10.1136/bmj.j909.

Hamwi, G. J. *Therapy: Changing Dietary Concepts.* New York: American Diabetes Association, 1964.

Holst, C., et al. "Alcohol Drinking Patterns and Risk of Diabetes: A Cohort Study of 70,551 Men and Women from the General Danish Population." *Diabetologia* 60, no. 10 (2017): 1941–1950. https://doi.org/10.1007/s00125-017-4359-3.

Joosten, M. M., et al. "Changes in Alcohol Consumption and Subsequent Risk of Type 2 Diabetes in Men." *Diabetes* 60, no. 1 (2011): 74–79. doi: 10.2337/db10-1052.

Wang, L., et al. "Alcohol Consumption, Weight Gain, and Risk of Becoming Overweight in Middle-Aged and Older Women." *Archives of Internal Medicine* 170, no. 5 (2010): 453–461. doi: 10.1001/archinternmed.2009.527.

Chapter 8

Blaise, B., et al. "Clearing the Brain's Cobwebs: The Role of Autophagy in Neuroprotection." *Current Neuropharmacology* 6, no. 2 (2008): 97–101. doi: 10.2174/157015908784533897.

Willette, A. A., et al. "Association of Insulin Resistance with Cerebral Glucose Uptake in Late Middle-Aged Adults at Risk for Alzheimer Disease." *JAMA Neurology* 72, no. 9 (2015): 1013–1020. doi:10.1001/jamaneurol.2015.0613.

Chapter 9

Boutcher, S. H. "High-Intensity Intermittent Exercise and Fat Loss." *Journal of Obesity* 2011 (2011): 868305. doi: 10.1155/2011/868305.

Robinson, M. M., et al. "Enhanced Protein Translation Underlies Improved Metabolic and Physical Adaptations to Different Exercise Training Modes in Young and Old Humans." *Cell Metabolism* 25, no. 3 (2017): 581–592. http://dx.doi.org/10.1016/j.cmet.2017.02.009.

Tucker, L. A. "Physical Activity and Telomere Length in U.S. Men and Women: An NHANES Investigation" *Preventive Medicine* 100 (2017): 145–151. https://doi.org/10.1016/j.ypmed.2017.04.027.

Van Proeyen, K. et al. "Training in the Fasted State Improves Glucose Tolerance during Fat-Rich Diet." *Journal of Physiology* 588, Pt 21 (2010): 4289–4302. doi: 10.1113/jphysiol.2010.196493.

Kumar, A., et al. "Role of Coenzyme Q10 (CoQ10) in Cardiac Disease, Hypertension, and Meniere-Like Syndrome." *Pharmacology & Therapeutics* 124, no. 3 (2009): 259–268. https://doi.org/10.1016/j.pharmthera.2009.07.003.

Singh U., et al. "Coenzyme Q10 Supplementation and Heart Failure." *Nutrition Reviews* 65, no. 6 Pt 1 (2007): 286–293. doi:10.1111/j.1753-4887.2007.tb00306.x.

Spindler, M., et al. "Coenzyme Q10 Effects in Neurodegenerative Disease." *Neuropsychiatric Disease and Treatment* 5 (2009): 597–610.

Ablon, G. "A 3-Month, Randomized, Double-Blind, Placebo-Controlled Study Evaluating the Ability of an Extra-Strength Marine Protein Supplement to Promote Hair Growth and Decrease Shedding in Women with Self-Perceived Thinning Hair." *Dermatology Research and Practice*, vol. 2015 (2015). doi:10.1155/2015/841570.

Clifford, T., et al. "The Potential Benefits of Red Beetroot Supplementation in Health and Disease." *Nutrients* 7, no. 4 (2015): 2801–2822. doi: 10.3390/nu7042801.

USDA Economic Research Service, "Potatoes and Tomatoes Are the Most Commonly Consumed Vegetables," https://www.ers.usda.gov/data-products/chart-gallery/gallery/chart-detail/?chartId=58340. Last updated Thursday, September 14, 2017.